NSC
Basic Life Support
for Health Care & Professional Rescuers
TEXTBOOK

12.5M1113

Interior design, layout and composition and cover design: Bending Design Inc.

DISCLAIMER

Although the information and recommendations contained in this publication have been compiled from sources believed to be reliable, the National Safety Council makes no guarantee as to, and assumes no responsibility for, the correctness, sufficiency, or completeness of such information or recommendations. Other or additional safety measures may be required under particular circumstances.

NATIONAL SAFETY COUNCIL MISSION STATEMENT

The National Safety Council saves lives by preventing injuries and deaths at work, in homes and communities, and on the roads through leadership, research, education and advocacy.

nsc.org

ISBN: 978-0-87912-306-2

About The National Safety Council

The National Safety Council® is a nonprofit organization whose mission is to save lives by preventing injuries and deaths at work, in homes and communities and on the road through leadership, research, education and advocacy. NSC advances this mission by partnering with businesses, government agencies, elected officials and the public to make an impact where the most preventable injuries and deaths occur, in areas such as distracted driving, teen driving, workplace safety and beyond the workplace, particularly in and near our homes.

Founded in 1913 and chartered by the U.S. Congress, the National Safety Council relies on research to determine optimal solutions to safety issues and directs its educational efforts to build awareness, provide training and share best practices. The Council recognizes organizations that have focused on safety as a critical part of their operational excellence with the Robert W. Campbell Award®, safety's most prestigious honor. NSC Congress & Expo is the world's largest annual event dedicated to safety, and Safety+Health® magazine is a leading source of occupational safety information. The World Health Organization named NSC the designated U.S. certification center for its Safe Communities America® Program. Each year, the Green Cross for Safety® Medal from NSC salutes a company with an outstanding safety record for its leadership in responsible citizenship and community service. Offering a variety of learning options, NSC is a leader in First Aid and Workplace Safety training and created the defensive driving course category where it remains the chief innovator.

The National Safety Council is committed to helping its members prevent unintentional injuries and deaths by providing knowledge and resources that enable them to reduce risks, engage employees, measure progress and continuously improve their safety management systems. With local Chapters and global networks, NSC is the leading advocate for safety and promotes June as National Safety Month.

Author Acknowledgements

Many National Safety Council staff and affiliates have contributed to the production of this book, and we would like to acknowledge the following people for their assistance:

Paul Satterlee, MD, for reviewing and providing oversight of content.

Goodman Research Inc., for program evaluation and recomendations for program improvement.

Tom Lochhaas, Editorial Services, for providing technical writing services.

Donna M. Siegfried, Senior Director, First Aid Programs, for providing vision and support.

Barbara Caracci, Director, Program Development and Training, for providing oversight of content, development and production.

Donna Fredenhagen, Product Manager, for providing marketing support.

Kathy Safranek, Project Administrator, for providing day-to-day assistance.

Roseann Solak, Manager, Product Development, for oversight management of development processes and design teams.

Pauline DePinto, Product Coordinator, for coordinating development and production.

Alice Spencer, Project Manager, for coordinating development and production.

The Council also recognizes with appreciation the many other NSC employees who devoted time to this project.

Reviewer Acknowledgements

Rebecca Gribben, BS, NREMT
Training Director
Advent Resource Management
Houston, TX

Patricia Jubinville, BS, EMT-P
Instructor Trainer
Safety Council of Central and Western New York
East Syracuse, NY

Deb Kaye, BS, NREMT
Director/Instructor EMS
Dakota County Technical College
Rosemount, MN

David Morgan, EMT, BS
Principal Trainer
Safety First
Newark, NJ

Robb Rehberg, PhD, ATC, CSCS, NREMT
Coordinator of Athletic Training Clinical Education
William Paterson University
Wayne, NJ

Jack Weberg
Instructor/Instructor Trainer
Arizona Chapter, National Safety Council
Phoenix, AZ

Table of Contents

Chapter 1 • Role of the Professional Rescuer

Professional rescuers work in a variety of settings and, as part of the Emergency Medical Services (EMS) system, have an important duty to give initial care to victims of injury or sudden illness. The basic life support skills described in this text are a key part of the emergency care professional rescuers provide. Professional rescuers need to understand their role within the EMS system and the legal issues involved in providing care. Professional rescuers also often have an important role in helping prevent injuries and common sudden illnesses.

Basic Life Support in Emergencies

Although professional rescuers may provide a wide variety of first aid for many types of injuries or **sudden illness**, care for life-threatening emergencies is most important. Two of the most serious threats to life are respiratory arrest and cardiac arrest. If the victim's breathing or heart stops, the victim has only minutes to live.

Basic life support (BLS) generally refers to care given when the victim's breathing or heart stops. Many things can cause breathing or the heart to stop. BLS is often needed for victims of:

- Heart attack
- Drowning
- Choking
- Other injuries or conditions that affect breathing or the heart

Heart attack is the single most common cause of death in emergency situations, followed by strokes and injuries. Each year the United States:

- More than 940,000 heart attacks occur, resulting in 150,000 deaths.
- Strokes result in 136,000 deaths.
- 128,200 people die from unintentional injuries.
- About 28 million visits are made to emergency departments because of unintentional injuries.

Table 1-1 lists the most common causes of injuries for which the victim went to a hospital emergency department in the most recent year for which data are available. **Table 1-2** lists the deaths resulting from the most common types of injuries in the most recent year for which data are available.

Table 1-1: Unintentional Injuries Treated in Hospital Emergency Departments in 2009

Falls	8,765,597
Struck by or against object	4,435,906
Overexertion	3,207,877
Motor vehicle occupants	2,643,652
Cut or pierced by object	1,997,752
Bites and stings (other than dog bites)	1,067,922
Other specified*	924,345
Unknown/unspecified	755,175
Poisoning (includes drug overdose)	708,318
Other transport**	602,434

Source: National Safety Council, "Injury Facts", 2012; data from NEISS All Injury Program, Office of Statistics and Programming, National Center for Injury Prevention and Control, Centers for Disease Control and Prevention, and Consumer Product Safety Commission.

* *Includes electric current, explosions, fireworks, radiation, animal scratch, etc.; excludes all causes listed in the table and bb/ pellet gunshot, drowning and near drowning, firearm gunshot, suffocation, machinery, natural and environmental conditions, pedestrians, and motorcyclists.*

** *Includes occupant of any transport vehicle other than a motor vehicle or motorcycle (e.g., airplane, rail car, boat, ATV, animal rider).*

Professional rescuers in any setting may give basic life support for victims of heart attack, stroke, choking, and many other kinds of life-threatening illnesses and injuries.

Professional Rescuers

A **professional rescuer** is a trained person who, in either an employment or a volunteer situation, has the responsibility to provide emergency care when needed. Following are some examples of professional rescuers **(Figure 1-1)**:

- Health care professionals: physicians, nurses, allied health professionals, EMTs, paramedics and emergency medical responders

- Firefighters

- Law enforcement, security and military personnel

- Park rangers, camp personnel, ski patrollers and lifeguards

- Responders in business, industry and farming

- Athletic trainers

Table 1-2: Deaths Due to Unintentional Injuries in 2010

Poisoning (includes drug overdose)	35,600
Motor vehicle incidents	35,500
Falls	28,000
Choking	4,700
Drowning	3,600
Fires, flames and smoke	3,100
Mechanical suffocation	1,900
All other unintentional injuries*	13,700

Source: National Safety Council, Injury Facts 2012; National Safety Council analysis of National Center for Health Statistics mortality data and Bureau of the Census population data.
* Includes natural heat and cold; firearms; struck by or against object; machinery; electric current; and air, water and rail transport.

- Airline and cruise ship personnel

- Public safety and search-and-rescue personnel

What individuals in these and other settings have in common is that they are called upon to give care to victims in an emergency. This responsibility generally includes:

1. Having the training to provide basic life support, and staying current in that training.

2. Accessing the EMS system to ensure a victim receives advanced medical care or rescue as quickly as possible when needed.

3. Ensuring the safety of the victim and others at the scene.

4. Managing the emergency scene and the victim until personnel with advanced training arrive and take over; assisting advanced personnel when needed.

A professional rescuer also should accept the responsibility to stay physically and mentally fit for these tasks; to review information and practice basic skills to stay proficient; and to act to prevent disease transmission to or from victims, others at the scene and oneself. It is important to maintain a healthy lifestyle to be prepared to act whenever needed, and to be able to control the stresses that may come with the job.

Being prepared, in addition to having basic life support skills, includes:

- Having confidence in your knowledge and skills.

- Readiness to act in a leadership role.

- Knowing where to access a first aid kit at any time.

- Knowing the telephone numbers for EMS (9-1-1 or local number in the United States), the U.S. Poison Control Center (800-222-1222), and other special services for your situation.

- Being able to access the EMS system (cell phone or radio).

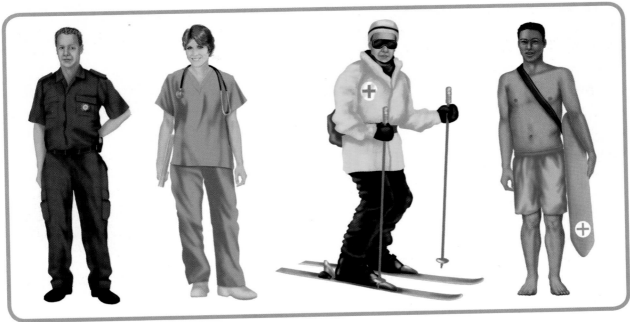

Figure 1-1 *Examples of professional rescuers.*

Professional Rescuer Versus Lay Rescuer

Professional rescuers include health care professionals and others who have a higher level of training than lay rescuers and perform more BLS skills. In addition, professional rescuers perform certain techniques in a different manner than most lay rescuers would perform them.

Professional rescuers follow the 2010 American Heart Association Guidelines for Cardiopulmonary Resuscitation and Emergency Cardiovascular Care recommendations for basic life support. **This text presents all BLS techniques as currently recommended for health care provider BLS rescuers.**

The EMS System

Professional rescuers are often the first step in the **emergency medical services (EMS) system**. In some cases a lay person may be first on the scene and may already be providing first aid. Someone already may have called 9-1-1. In many cases you will be the first professional to respond to the emergency, called by someone at the scene or by the EMS **dispatcher**. As such, you often are the first link in the process for ensuring the victim gets whatever help is needed.

The EMS system in the United States is a comprehensive network of professionals linked together to provide appropriate levels of medical care for victims of injury or sudden illness.* As a professional rescuer, your role in the system, in addition to caring for the victim until seen by more advanced caregivers, is to make sure the EMS system responds as soon as possible. If you are not a member of a responding EMS team, call 9-1-1 (or your local or company emergency number) and, in most communities in the United States, help will arrive within minutes.

The EMS system includes a number of different professionals with different levels of training and responsibilities.

Legal Issues

Professional rescuers should understand their legal obligations for providing emergency care and other legal issues. Following accepted guidelines

*The term **sudden illness** is generally used to describe a medical emergency that occurs suddenly and requires basic life support or first aid until the person receives more advanced medical attention. This term will be used throughout this text.

EMS PROFESSIONALS

Dispatcher

A 9-1-1 call is usually received by an EMS dispatcher. This person is trained in obtaining information and determining what emergency personnel and equipment will likely be needed. The EMS dispatcher then sends the appropriate EMS unit to the scene.

Emergency Medical Responder (EMR)

The first professional with BLS training to arrive at the scene of a medical emergency is often an **emergency medical responder** (formerly called a first responder). The EMR generally takes over care of the victim from a lay person who may be giving first aid or from anyone with less training. The EMR also gathers any information concerning the victim, may control the scene or direct others to do so, and in some instances prepares for the arrival of an ambulance. In a health care setting a professional rescuer may provide emergency care until a physician, nurse or other health care professional with a higher level of training takes over. In an out-of-hospital setting, emergency care may be given until emergency medical technicians arrive with an ambulance.

Emergency Medical Technicians (EMT) and Paramedics

In an out-of-hospital emergency, **Emergency Medical Technicians** and/or Advanced EMTs and Paramedics usually arrive in an ambulance. They take over the medical care of the victim, give necessary medical care at the scene, and

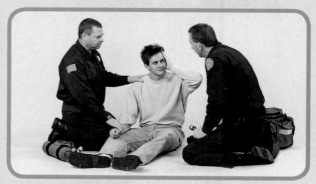

Figure 1-2 *EMTs take over the prehospital care of a victim.*

transport the victim for advanced medical care **(Figure 1-2)**. EMTs with different levels of training perform different medical treatments. Paramedics have the highest level of training.

Medical Director

The medical director is a physician within the EMS system who oversees the care given by EMTs and some EMRs. The medical director establishes protocols for medical care to be given to victims at the scene and is available for consultation by radio or telephone to EMTs giving care.

Hospitals and Specialized Centers

EMRs and EMTs provide prehospital care before and during the transport of the victim to a hospital. Depending on the medical care needed and facilities in the area, the victim receives care from physicians in a hospital emergency department or a specialized center such as a trauma center, burn center or pediatric center.

helps ensure you will not be found legally liable if a victim does not fully recover. Always follow these general principles:

1. Act only as you are trained to act.
2. Obtain a victim's consent before giving care.
3. Do not move a victim unnecessarily.
4. Call for more advanced medical help.
5. Keep giving care until relieved by a professional with a higher level of training.

Duty to Act

As a professional, you have a **duty to act** to care for a victim of a medical emergency. You have accepted this responsibility as a dimension of your job, and failing to care for a victim while you are on the job can make you legally liable.

State laws vary regarding your legal responsibility to act when off the job. Ask your instructor or research your state's laws to learn whether you are obligated to give care at an emergency scene you encounter as a private citizen. Note, however, that even as a private citizen, once you begin to give care in an emergency, you have accepted and taken on an obligation to continue giving care until someone with equal or greater training takes over. Abandoning a victim in this situation could lead to an injury or illness worsening, disability or death for which you may be legally liable.

Consent

Before giving care, you must have the victim's **consent**. Touching another person without consent is a criminal action called battery. Consent may be either expressed or implied.

Expressed consent means the victim explicitly gives you permission to provide emergency care. Tell the victim who you are and that you have had basic life support training, and say what you want to do to help. The victim should understand that you are asking for consent, not stating what you plan to do regardless of what the victim wishes. A victim who is responsive (awake and alert) and able to communicate must give you expressed consent by telling you it is okay or by nodding agreement. With an injured or ill child, a parent or guardian who is present must give expressed consent.

If the victim is unresponsive, or a child's parent or guardian is not present and cannot be reached quickly enough for consent, then you have **implied consent** to give care in an emergency. You can assume, unless there is evidence to the contrary, that the person would, if able, consent to receiving care for a life-threatening condition.

Refusal of Consent

Most competent victims in a medical emergency will give consent when they understand the importance of the care you are offering. **Competent** means the person is able to understand what is happening and the implications of his or her decision. A victim may not be competent because of intoxication, the influence of a drug, or altered mental status caused by an injury or illness.

In rare instances, a competent victim may refuse your care when you seek consent. The person may have religious reasons, may be afraid, may not trust you or may have some other reason. Regardless of the reason, a competent adult has the right to refuse medical care, even care that has already begun, and you must not force care in this situation. The victim's refusal may be expressed through words, by shaking the head or signaling you to stop, or by trying to push you away. If this happens, follow these guidelines:

- To protect yourself legally, make sure someone else at the scene sees or hears the victim's refusal to accept your care, and document it as soon as you can.

- Make sure 9-1-1 or advanced medical personnel have been called, even though the victim may seem to refuse all care. The victim might accept treatment from another medical professional.

- Keep talking to the victim, who may change his or her mind. Explain that you respect his or her right to refuse care but ask the person to reconsider. Explain what may happen if the victim does not receive care.

Advance Directives

An advance directive is a specific form of refusing care. An **advance directive**, sometimes called a living will, is a legal document, signed by an individual (often a terminally ill person) and his or her doctor, that identifies what medical care the person will or will not accept. Often this means the ill person has chosen not to be resuscitated if his or her heart and breathing stop. A written statement of this is called a **Do Not Resuscitate**

(DNR) order. This would mean, for example, that the person does not want to receive CPR or defibrillation. Most terminally ill patients with DNR orders are in a hospital or nursing home, but many are at home. Because of the legal issues involved, a professional rescuer must be certain about the written DNR document before deciding not to give basic life support. Statements by a family member about what the victim would want, for example, cannot be used to withhold lifesaving care. A professional rescuer working in a health care facility where DNR orders are more common should follow the facility's policy for providing or withholding specific kinds of care. Note that a DNR order that refers to resuscitation does not apply to other kinds of treatment, which you should still provide.

Scope of Practice

As noted earlier, professional rescuers should give only the care they have been trained to give. The set of basic life support skills learned in this course, along with skills from other recognized courses, are part of your **scope of practice**. Acting outside your scope of practice, such as trying to do something you have seen others do but have not been trained to do yourself, may make you legally liable for the results of your actions.

Standard of Care

Standard of care refers generally to how you give care and what others with your same training would do in a similar situation. Standards are generally determined by professional organizations, laws and other recognized authorities. You will learn the standards of care for basic life support in this course. Performing care in a way that does not meet the standards could result in the victim's injury or illness becoming worse, and could make you legally liable.

Negligence and Abandonment

Not following accepted standards of care when giving care is called **negligence**. In cases of negligence an injured party may sue to recover financial damages for the result of your actions.

You may be found guilty of negligence only if three conditions are met:

1. You have a duty to act.
2. You breach that duty (by not acting or by acting incorrectly).
3. Your actions or inaction causes injury or damages (including physical injury or pain).

Examples of negligent actions could include moving a victim unnecessarily, doing something you have not been trained to do or failing to give care as you have been trained to do.

Abandonment is a specific type of negligence. Once you begin giving emergency care, you must not stop until another professional with equal or greater training takes over. If you leave the victim and the injury or illness becomes worse, you may be found guilty of abandonment. Note that abandonment is different from justified instances of stopping care, such as if you are exhausted and unable to continue or you are in imminent danger because of hazards at the scene.

Confidentiality

While giving care, you may learn private information about the victim. You should not share that information with anyone other than health care professionals caring for the victim. Although state laws vary in terms of precise definitions regarding violation of privacy, **confidentiality** is the general principle that states you should not give out any information about a victim to anyone except for those caring for the victim.

Documentation

In most cases, your employer requires that you document actions you take in an emergency. Most agencies and facilities use specific forms you must complete shortly after giving emergency care. Be aware that any written record may become legal evidence, and document the incident fully and in factual detail. Sign and date this document and, when appropriate, include the names or signatures of witnesses.

Good Samaritan Laws

Most states have **Good Samaritan laws** designed to encourage people to help others in an emergency without worrying about being sued. These laws vary from state to state, but in general they are designed to protect people who give care in an emergency. Ask your instructor about your state's specific Good Samaritan law, which may have provisions about providing emergency care on or off the job.

Good Samaritan laws do not provide blanket protection, however. You are legally protected only when you follow standards of care, obtain consent and meet the other legal criteria previously described.

Preventing Emergencies

Professional rescuers are often in a position to help prevent emergencies in the settings in which they work. Injuries commonly occur when someone fails to prevent them by not following accepted safety standards or not using common sense. It is beyond the scope of this book to cover the specific steps that can be taken to prevent injuries in all settings, but professional rescuers – with a little research and observation – can learn what the risks are in their own work settings and how to help others prevent injuries and other emergencies. Following are some general guidelines for injury prevention:

- In your workplace and home, take steps to prevent fires, accidental poisonings and other injuries. Look for hazards and correct them.

- In the workplace, always follow safety procedures required by the Occupational Safety and Health Administration (OSHA). If you have received safety training, use it. It takes only one lapse from a safety procedure to lose a life.

- Use common sense when driving or engaging in activities involving injury risks. As Table 1-1 shows, the majority of injuries seen in hospital emergency departments result from falls, being struck by or against an object, overexertion, motor vehicle crashes, or being cut or pierced by an object.

As with injuries, many sudden illness emergencies can be prevented. A healthy lifestyle helps prevent heart attack, stroke, hypertension, diabetes and other diseases that may result in life-threatening medical emergencies. A healthy lifestyle begins with avoiding the well-known **risk factors** that contribute to these diseases. Stop smoking, eat a diet low in fats and sugars, exercise regularly, control your weight, and learn to manage stress. Chapter 3 describes these strategies for healthful living in more detail.

Coping With The Stress of Emergencies

Emergencies are stressful, especially when the victim does not survive. Not every victim can be saved. Injuries, illness or circumstances are often beyond our control. Particularly stressful emergencies include those that involve multiple victims, children, victims of abuse or neglect, or death or injury of a co-worker or friend.

It is normal to have a strong emotional reaction during and immediately after a stressful emergency. Often this reaction gradually diminishes with time, but in some cases the stress remains and problems may result. Stress can cause irritability when interacting with others, difficulty sleeping, problems concentrating, general anxiety or depression, and even physical symptoms. If you recognize that you are feeling or behaving differently after experiencing a traumatic emergency, you may need help coping.

- Remind yourself that your reaction is normal, that we all need help sometimes.

- Talk to others: family members, co-workers, other professional rescuers, local emergency responders or your own health care provider. (Do not breach confidentiality of the victim.)

- Many organizations and facilities have a formal program involving a **critical incident stress debriefing**, which generally includes group discussions and the guidance of professionals trained in stress reduction. Do not hesitate to use such a program.

- Do not be afraid or reluctant to seek professional help. Many employers have an employee assistance program or member assistance program that can help or make a referral. Or, ask your health care provider for a referral.

Conclusion

Professional rescuers work in a wide variety of settings but share the responsibility of giving emergency care, including basic life support, for injuries and sudden illness. Professional rescuers must clearly understand their responsibilities to be prepared for emergencies, their role within the EMS system and the legal issues involved in giving care.

Review Questions

1. What is the single most common cause of death in emergency situations?
   a. Vehicular accidents
   b. Strokes
   c. Burns
   d. Heart attacks

2. As a professional rescuer you have a legal obligation to –
   a. do anything possible for victims.
   b. give care as you have been trained.
   c. risk your life if necessary to save another.
   d. care for a victim only until your work shift ends.

3. In which of the following circumstances do you NOT have consent to give care?
   a. An alert victim refuses care for religious reasons.
   b. The victim is a child without a parent or guardian present.
   c. The victim is unconscious.
   d. A victim nods consent but does not actually give consent aloud.

4. Which of the following actions might be determined to be negligence?
   a. When off duty, you forget to carry your cell phone and happen to be the first at an accident scene.
   b. While you are correctly providing CPR to a victim in cardiac arrest, two ribs are cracked.
   c. You use a new burn treatment you read about in a professional journal but were not trained to perform.
   d. Your pen runs out of ink when you are filling out an incident report, and you do not have another pen with you.

5. If you still feel very stressed several days after providing care in an emergency, you should NOT –
   a. tell your supervisor.
   b. talk to family members.
   c. keep your feelings to yourself.
   d. see your health care provider.

Case Scenario

Mark Johnson, a park ranger trained as a professional rescuer, and his partner encounter a lone hiker in a trail parking lot. The man is more than 60 years old and overweight. The man is leaning against his car, breathing fast, sweating heavily and rubbing his chest with one hand. Mark stops to ask him if he is okay, and the man, short of breath and speaking with difficulty, says he is okay but too out of shape for the hike he just took. He grimaces as if in pain, and Mark asks if he is feeling chest pain. "It's just indigestion," the man says, and waves Mark off. Mark realizes, however, that the man could be having a heart attack.

1. Because the man has refused Mark's offer to help, what should Mark do?
   a. Back away, but keep watching the man in case he collapses, in which case Mark has implied consent to give treatment.
   b. Nothing. He should go on about his work, and later when in the office should write a report stating that the man refused care.
   c. Take the man's car keys away and call for an ambulance.
   d. Keep talking to the man and explain that he might be having a heart attack, which could become very serious if he ignores it; offer to call for help.

While Mark is talking to him, the man suddenly clutches his chest and collapses to the ground, unresponsive. Mark tells his partner to call 9-1-1 as he positions the man to assess his condition.

2. As a professional rescuer, what is Mark now legally obligated to do?
   a. Provide care as he has been trained to do.
   b. Respect the man's earlier refusal of care but stay with him until EMS personnel take over.
   c. Contact a family member for permission to care for him.
   d. Nothing – he has no legal obligations in this situation.

Chapter 2 • Victim Assessment and Basic Life Support

Basic life support skills are used to resuscitate a victim who is not breathing adequately or does not have a heartbeat, or to keep the victim alive until advanced medical care is available. Care of the victim begins with the initial assessment of the victim's responsiveness and normal breathing.

Overview of Basic Life Support

Of all injuries and illnesses, the most immediate threats to life are those involving the airway, breathing or circulation of blood. When a problem occurs in any of these areas, the victim's body cells do not receive enough oxygen and brain cells begin to die within minutes. The victim needs immediate basic life support to survive. The goals of basic life support are to:

- Resuscitate the victim if possible by restoring circulation, an open airway and normal breathing.

- Ensure the victim receives advanced medical care by calling for help.

- Keep the victim alive until he or she receives advanced medical care.

- Prevent the victim's condition from getting worse.

Basic life support generally consists of several types of care often given together and collectively called **resuscitation**. A victim who is not responsive and not breathing normally is presumed to be in cardiac arrest, and therefore needs chest compressions to circulate the blood so that some oxygen reaches vital organs. A professional rescuer also provides rescue breaths to move oxygen into the lungs to circulate in the blood. The combination of chest compressions and rescue breaths is called **cardiopulmonary resuscitation (CPR)**. A victim who is not breathing adequately because of an airway obstruction, or choking, also needs care to clear the airway to allow either natural breathing or rescue breathing. Finally,

a victim whose heart may be in a condition called ventricular fibrillation, which is common after heart attacks and other situations, may benefit from an electrical shock given by an automated external defibrillator (AED) to restore a regular heartbeat.

The next three chapters describe these dimensions of basic life support in detail. This chapter discusses how to begin the process of basic life support by assessing the victim to detect these immediate threats to life.

Differences Among Adults, Children and Infants

Because of size and other differences, there are some distinctions in how BLS skills are used with adults, children and infants. These age-dependent differences result from anatomical and physiological differences in the human body at different ages. Differences in BLS techniques are described throughout the next three BLS chapters. Standard age groups for BLS are defined in the following way. Remember these age categories in reference to all BLS techniques:

- An *infant* is up to 1 year old.

- A *child* for purposes of all BLS skills (including rescue breathing and CPR) is 1 year up to the onset of adolescence or puberty (as determined by the occurrence of secondary sex characteristics, such as the presence of armpit hair in boys or breast development in girls); for AED only, a child means ages 1 to 8.

- An *adult* for all BLS skills except for AED means at or past puberty; for AED only, adult means older than 8.

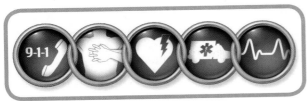

Figure 2-1 *Cardiac chain of survival.*

The Cardiac Chain of Survival

Although BLS includes care given to any victim whose breathing or circulation stops, cardiac arrest victims are a common type of victim needing BLS. **Cardiac arrest** refers to a sudden stop in the beating of the heart.

To recognize the need for quick actions to save the lives of cardiac arrest victims, the Citizen CPR Foundation created the concept of the **cardiac chain of survival (Figure 2-1)**. This chain has five crucial links:

1. ***Immediate recognition of the cardiac arrest and activation of the emergency response system***. Recognize that a victim whose heart has stopped needs help immediately! It is also important that you recognize the signs and symptoms of a potential life-threatening condition such as heart attack or stroke in a responsive person (see Chapter 3). Do not wait until a person becomes unresponsive to start the chain of events needed to keep him or her alive. Call 9-1-1 and get help on the way. The victim needs early access to advanced medical care.

2. ***Early CPR with emphasis on chest compressions***. For a victim without a pulse, start cardiopulmonary resuscitation (CPR) immediately. This helps keep the brain and other vital organs supplied with oxygen until the AED arrives.

3. ***Rapid defibrillation***. An AED, usually present in health care agencies as well as in many public settings and workplaces, can help get the heart beating normally again after a cardiac arrest. Send someone right away to get the AED.

4. ***Effective advanced life support***. The sooner the victim is treated by advanced emergency

care professionals, the better the chance for survival. You can help make sure the victim reaches this link in the chain by acting immediately with the earlier links.

5. ***Integrated post-cardiac arrest care***. Following early care, the victim needs continued, integrated medical care by a team of medical professionals, typically within a hospital or other advanced medical center.

Call First/Call Fast

In any situation in which you recognize that a victim of injury or illness is unresponsive and not breathing normally, if someone else is present at the scene, have that person call for help immediately. Shout for anyone who may hear you, and have them get help or call 9-1-1 and go for an AED.

If you are alone, however, you need to decide whether to call immediately or to first begin to provide care for the victim. The following guidelines are based on determinations of what is usually needed for victims in different circumstances.

When alone, as a general rule your rescue response should depend on the most likely cause of the victim's problem. **Call first** for a victim of any age seen to collapse suddenly. These victims are more likely to be in cardiac arrest and to require defibrillation. Calling EMS immediately starts the process of getting an AED to the victim sooner.

If an adult victim is found unresponsive and not breathing normally, you should still **call first** for help and an AED before providing CPR because the most likely cause is cardiac arrest. With a young child or infant victim, however, an airway obstruction is a more likely cause, so **call fast** after providing about 5 cycles of CPR (about 2 minutes).

For unresponsive victims whose circumstances suggest a likely asphyxial arrest, such as a drowning victim or a victim with an airway obstruction, **call fast**. Give about 5 cycles of CPR (about 2 minutes) before stopping to call EMS.

The Initial Assessment

When you recognize that an emergency is occurring, first check that it is safe to approach the victim, and then quickly assess the victim for immediate threats to life. This is called the **initial assessment**.

Scene Safety

In many emergency situations, hazards may be present at the scene that threaten your own safety. Always check the scene before approaching a victim; you must be safe yourself if you are to help another. Look for hazards such as smoke or flames, spilled chemicals or fumes, downed electrical wires, traffic dangers, and so on. If the scene is dangerous and you cannot safely approach the victim, **stay away and call for help**. The 9-1-1 dispatcher will send a crew with the appropriate training and equipment to safely reach and care for the victim.

Checking the Victim

When you first reach the victim, quickly check him or her in the position found. Spinal and other injuries could be made worse by moving the victim unnecessarily. If the victim seems unresponsive, check by tapping the victim on the shoulder and shouting, "Are you okay?" A victim who can speak, cough or make other sounds is breathing and has a heartbeat, and may not need to be moved. At the same time you are checking for responsiveness, look for normal breathing. An unresponsive victim who is only gasping is not breathing normally and needs basic life support. Ensure a call for help is made.

If the victim is unresponsive and not breathing normally, then you need to position the victim on his or her back. Check quickly for a pulse. Then begin CPR with chest compressions (if no pulse) or provide rescue breathing (if not breathing or not breathing normally but has a pulse).

If the victim can speak or cough, then he or she has an open airway, is breathing, and has a beating heart. This victim should then quickly be checked for life-threatening bleeding and other injuries.

Except when a spinal injury is suspected, a victim who is unresponsive but who is breathing normally should be put in the recovery position, as described later.

Precautions with Spinal Injuries

If it is necessary to position a non-breathing unresponsive victim with a potential spinal injury, support the head in line with the body as you move the victim. This usually requires the help of others. If the victim is lying face down, with the help of one or two other people, roll the victim onto his or her back, supporting the head through the entire move **(Figure 2-2)**.

Checking Circulation

Lay rescuers trained in CPR are taught to begin CPR with chest compressions immediately for an unresponsive victim who is not breathing normally. Health care and professional rescuers who are trained to check for a **pulse** should check for a pulse before beginning chest compressions – but must do this very quickly. It is critical not to use more than 10 seconds to feel for the victim's pulse; unless a pulse is clearly found in that time, start chest compressions immediately. If an obvious pulse is found, then begin rescue breathing immediately, as described in the following chapter.

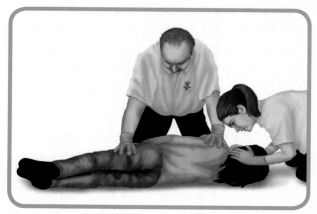

Figure 2-2 *Positioning an unresponsive victim who is not breathing normally and who has a potential spinal injury.*

If a pulse is not found, the victim is presumed to be in cardiac arrest. If the victim's heart has stopped, vital organs are not receiving enough oxygen to sustain life.

Special note for previously trained rescuers. Prior to October 2010, rescuers were taught BLS care in an ABC series of actions (open airway, give breaths, and start compressions). With more research, the protocol has changed to emphasize beginning with compressions (a CAB order). If you originally learned CPR using the ABC order, be sure to focus now on the importance of beginning with chest compressions following a very *quick* pulse check.

It takes training to be able to effectively and quickly locate a pulse **(Figure 2-3)**. To check the pulse in an adult, use the **carotid pulse** in the neck. Holding the victim's forehead with one hand to keep the airway open, put the index and middle fingers of your other hand on the side of the victim's neck nearest you. Find the Adam's apple and then slide your fingertips toward you and down the victim's neck to the groove at the side of the neck. Pressing gently, feel for a pulse for at least 5 but not more than 10 seconds.

In a child, check either the carotid or the **femoral pulse**. The femoral pulse is located in the center of the groin crease.

To check the pulse in an infant, use the **brachial pulse** in the inside of the upper arm instead of the carotid or femoral pulse. With one hand on the infant's forehead to maintain head position for an open airway, put the fingers of your other hand about midway between the shoulder and elbow on the inside of the arm and press gently, feeling for no more than 10 seconds.

Lack of a definite pulse along with the absence of normal breathing signifies the heart has stopped or is not beating effectively enough to circulate blood. If the victim lacks a pulse and is not breathing normally, start CPR and call for an AED to be brought to the scene, as described in Chapters 3 and 4.

Checking for Severe Bleeding

The initial assessment of a victim focuses on immediate threats to life. Unresponsiveness and not breathing normally, as noted above, are both life-threatening emergencies requiring immediate care and calling for help. Although care given for severe bleeding is not considered basic life support, it too is an immediate threat to life – call for help immediately and care for the victim as you have been trained.

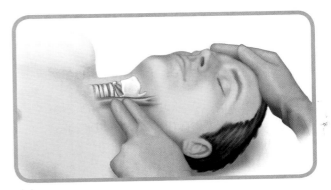

(a)

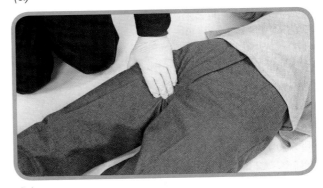

(b)

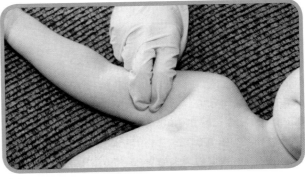

(c)

Fig 2-3 *Checking the pulse. (a) Carotid pulse. (b) Femoral pulse. (c) Brachial pulse.*

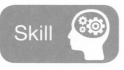

Skill — Initial Assessment

1 Check for responsiveness and normal breathing. Tap the victim's shoulder and shout, "Are you okay?"

2 If the victim is unresponsive, call 9-1-1. If the victim is unresponsive and not breathing, also call for an AED and provide basic life support.

3 If the victim is not breathing, check for a pulse for no longer than 10 seconds. If no pulse, start CPR with chest compressions; if a pulse is detected, start rescue breathing.

4 If the victim is breathing, check for severe bleeding and other threats to life.

5 Care for any life-threatening conditions before continuing to check the victim and provide other care.

The Secondary Assessment

If the initial assessment of the victim reveals any life-threatening conditions, immediately begin care for those conditions. Only if it is clear that the victim does not have a life-threatening condition, including bleeding, do you move on to the **secondary assessment** to check for additional injuries or signs of a sudden illness requiring care.

The secondary assessment includes obtaining a history from the victim or others present about what happened, what may have led to the illness or injury, other signs and symptoms, and so on. It also may include a physical examination of the victim to find injuries or other problems requiring care that are not immediately apparent. These skills are typically taught in first aid and emergency medical responder courses.

The Recovery Position

An unresponsive victim who does not have a breathing or circulation problem, and who is not suspected to have a spinal injury, should be put in the HAINES **recovery position**. (HAINES stands for High Arm IN Endangered Spine.) This position is used for several reasons:

- It helps keep the airway open so you do not need to maintain the head tilt–chin lift position.

- It allows fluids to drain from the mouth so the victim does not choke on blood, vomit or other fluids.

- It prevents the victim from inhaling stomach contents if he or she vomits.

If possible, unless this could worsen the victim's injury, put the victim on his or her left side. Because of anatomical differences in the body, the left side has more benefits for protecting the victim. On the left side, vomiting is delayed, the movement of poison into the small intestine is slower, and in a pregnant woman there is less pressure on the vena cava, the large vein of the heart. See "Skill: HAINES Recovery Position" on page 15 for the steps for moving an unresponsive breathing adult or child into the recovery position. **Figure 2-4** shows how to hold an infant in the recovery position.

Once the victim is in the recovery position, continue to monitor his or her breathing while waiting for advanced help to arrive.

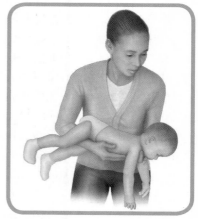

Figure 2-4 *Infant held in recovery position.*

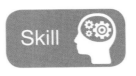

HAINES Recovery Position

1 Extend the victim's arm that is farther from you above his or her head.

2 Position the victim's other arm across the chest.

3 Bend the victim's nearer leg at the knee.

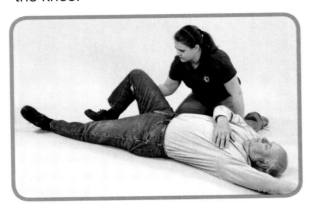

4 Put your forearm under the victim's shoulder with your hand around the back of the neck to support the head and neck.

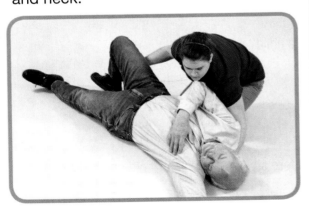

5 Carefully roll the victim away from you by pushing on the victim's flexed knee and lifting with your forearm while your hand stabilizes the head and neck. The victim's head is now supported on the raised arm.

6 While continuing to support the head and neck, position the victim's hand palm-down with fingers under the armpit of the raised arm, with forearm flat on the surface at 90 degrees to the body.

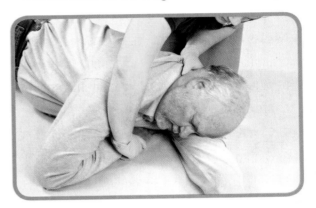

7 Bend both legs so the victim's position is stabilized.

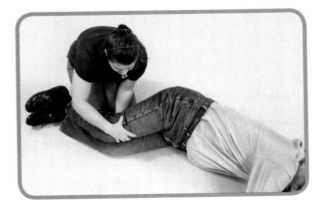

8 With the victim now in position, check the airway and open the mouth to allow drainage.

Conclusion

Care for a victim with a potentially life-threatening condition begins with the initial assessment: checking for unresponsiveness, lack of normal breathing and other threats to life. Life-threatening problems must be treated immediately. The basic life support skills used to care for these problems are described in the following chapters.

Review Questions

1. Which pulse should be checked in an infant who is not breathing?
   a. Carotid pulse *Adult & child*
   b. Brachial pulse *Infant*
   c. Posterior tibial pulse
   d. Radial pulse

2. Assess an adult victim for responsiveness by –
   a. tapping the shoulder and shouting, "Are you okay?"
   b. pinching the cheek between thumb and forefinger.
   c. checking for pupil reactions to light.
   d. checking skin for normal color and temperature.

3. Advantages of the recovery position include –
   a. it lowers the victim's blood pressure.
   b. it allows fluids to drain from the mouth.
   c. it helps prevent shock.
   d. it helps the heart maintain a normal rhythm.

4. For the purposes of BLS, when does an infant become a child?
   a. At 6 months
   b. At 1 year
   c. At 15 lbs
   d. At 25 lbs

5. For which victim should you provide 5 cycles of CPR before stopping to call for help and an AED?
   a. An adult seen to collapse suddenly
   b. An adult found unresponsive of unknown causes
   c. An infant found unresponsive
   d. An older adult in any circumstance

Case Scenario

You and your partner arrive at the scene, where an elderly gentleman says he is experiencing chest pains. As you enter, you see the elderly gentleman stand up from his chair and then collapse on the floor onto his side.

1. What action should you take first?

   a. Open his airway and listen for breathing.

   b. Check him for responsiveness and normal breathing.

   c. Take his pulse.

   d. Move him into the recovery position.

2. He does not respond and is not breathing. You quickly position him on his back. What should you do next?

   a. Start giving rescue breaths.

   b. Look in his mouth for a foreign object.

   c. Thump his chest with your fist as hard as you can.

   d. Check for a pulse in no more than 10 seconds.

3. While you are taking this action (above), your partner should be –

   a. calling for additional help and an AED if you do not already have one at the scene.

   b. giving chest compressions.

   c. turning the victim into the recovery position.

   d. listening at the victim's mouth for sounds of breathing.

4. You do not detect a pulse. An AED is on its way. You and your partner should now –

   a. start CPR with chest compressions.

   b. start CPR with rescue breaths.

   c. check again for a pulse.

   d. put the victim in the recovery position until the AED arrives.

Chapter 3 • Cardiovascular Emergencies and Cardiopulmonary Resuscitation (CPR)

Cardiac and respiratory emergencies are among the most serious threats to life. Basic life support is needed for a victim whose heartbeat or breathing has stopped or is inadequate. Rescue breaths are given to oxygenate the blood in someone whose breathing is inadequate or has stopped. If the victim's heart has stopped beating normally, chest compressions also are given to circulate blood to vital organs. Rescue breathing combined with chest compressions is called **cardiopulmonary resuscitation (CPR)**. This chapter discusses cardiac and respiratory emergencies and the basic life support care given victims with these threats to life.

Cardiovascular Disease and Emergencies

Cardiovascular disease includes diseases of the heart and blood vessels. Common diseases include **hypertension** (high blood pressure), **atherosclerosis** (narrowing and blockage of the arteries often caused by **high cholesterol** levels) and **coronary artery disease** (blockage of the coronary arteries to the heart muscle). Cardiovascular diseases raise the risk of cardiovascular emergencies such as stroke and heart attack, which, along with cancer, are two of the top three causes of death. Much cardiovascular disease can be prevented.

Stroke

A **stroke**, also called a cerebrovascular accident (CVA), is an interruption of blood flow to a part of the brain, killing nerve cells and affecting the victim's functioning. Stroke is a cardiovascular disease that, like heart attack, may be caused by atherosclerosis. About 800,000 Americans a year have a stroke, resulting in about 137,000 deaths and disabling many stroke victims who survive. Strokes are more common in older adults.

A stroke victim needs medical help immediately to decrease the chance of permanent damage. Therefore it is very important to be able to identify stroke in a victim.

Signs and Symptoms of Stroke

Stroke generally causes a sudden weakness or numbness in the face, arm or leg, especially on one side; sudden confusion; difficulty understanding speech; and difficulty speaking or swallowing, possibly with vision problems in one or both eyes. The victim may have trouble walking, dizziness, or loss of balance or coordination. The victim may experience a sudden, severe headache of unknown cause, and may have changing levels of responsiveness. The exact signs and symptoms occurring in a stroke victim depend on the site in the brain where an artery is blocked, and therefore vary somewhat. The victim's signs and symptoms may mistakenly be attributed to some other condition that affects responsiveness. A screening assessment, such as the Cincinnati Prehospital Stroke Scale, should be used to accurately identify a stroke.

THE CINCINNATI PREHOSPITAL STROKE SCALE

The more quickly stroke is recognized, the more quickly the victim can be given appropriate prehospital care and rushed to a stroke center or other appropriate treatment center. The **Cincinnati Prehospital Stroke Scale (CPSS)** is widely used to identify stroke. The CPSS uses three simple assessments:

1. Ask the victim to smile.

2. Ask the victim to raise both arms out in front of the body.

3. Ask the victim to repeat this sentence: "You can't teach an old dog new tricks."

A victim experiencing a stroke typically manifests these signs:

1. Only one side of the face makes a smile; the other side seems to "droop."

2. One arm does not move or drifts away from the position in front of the body.

3. The victim slurs words, uses the wrong words or cannot speak at all.

In an out-of-hospital setting, also try to learn when the signs and symptoms first occurred. Ask family members or others present at the scene as well as the victim. This information is important for the EMS treatment of the victim.

Care for Stroke

The most important thing to do for a stroke victim is to access advanced medical care. Call for help within a health care facility, or in an out-of-hospital setting call 9-1-1 immediately. Drugs can often minimize the effects of a stroke – but only if administered very soon afterward. Tell the dispatcher you believe the victim has had a stroke and describe his or her signs and symptoms. Take note of the time when signs and symptoms began. Be calming and reassuring to the victim, who often does not understand what has happened and is confused or fearful. Have the victim lie down on his or her back with head and shoulders slightly raised; this is often called the "stroke position" **(Figure 3-1)**. Loosen a constrictive collar. If necessary, turn the victim's head to the side to allow saliva or vomit to drain. Administer **supplemental oxygen** to the victim if it is available and you are trained in its use (Appendix B). Monitor the victim and be prepared for vomiting and to give BLS if needed. Move an unresponsive victim into the recovery position and ensure the airway remains open.

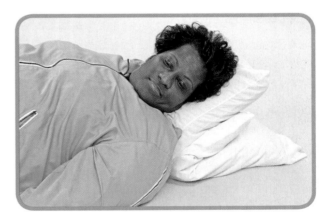

Figure 3-1 *Stroke position.*

Transient Ischemic Attack (TIA)

A **transient ischemic attack (TIA)**, sometimes called a mini-stroke, is a temporary interruption to blood flow in an artery in the brain. A TIA produces signs and symptoms similar to those of a stroke, except they usually disappear within a few minutes. Because a person who experiences a TIA is at a high risk for a stroke, advanced care should always be given to a victim who exhibits the signs and symptoms of stroke, even if they seem mild or soon disappear.

PREVENTING CARDIOVASCULAR DISEASE

A risk factor is anything that makes it more likely that a person will develop a particular disease. Following are known risk factors for cardiovascular disease:

Risk factors that cannot be changed

- Increasing age
- Race
- Hereditary factors

Preventable risk factors

- Smoking
- High cholesterol levels
- High blood pressure
- Physical inactivity
- Obesity and overweight
- Stress

Even though some risk factors cannot be changed, it is important to understand how they increase your risk of cardiovascular disease. In general, the risks of these diseases rise with increasing age. Men are more likely to have cardiovascular disease – although the rates are also high in women, who should not feel immune to heart attacks or other cardiovascular problems. African-Americans generally have a higher prevalence of high blood pressure than Caucasian Americans and therefore have a greater risk for cardiovascular disease. Hereditary factors such as a family history of heart disease also can increase one's risk.

If you know that your risk for cardiovascular disease is high because of risk factors beyond your control, this makes it all the more important to prevent those risk factors you can control. Risk factors often have an additive effect: the more risk factors you have, the higher your danger overall for developing disease.

Prevention of cardiovascular disease involves eliminating or minimizing risk factors by adopting a healthy lifestyle. In general, this means:

- Not using tobacco
- Eating healthy foods to prevent overweight, help lower cholesterol levels and blood pressure, and help prevent diabetes
- Maintaining low cholesterol levels, with medication when appropriate
- Controlling high blood pressure with diet, exercise, weight control and medication if needed
- Getting sufficient regular exercise to help prevent overweight, high blood pressure, diabetes and stress
- Preventing or managing stress

Notice how these risk factors are interrelated. For example, inactivity puts one at risk for being overweight, and weight control also helps prevent hypertension and manage stress. Eating well also helps prevent overweight and control blood pressure. Interrelated risk factors are sometimes referred to as a "constellation" of factors. Similarly, maintaining good cardiovascular health should focus not on one or two individual factors but on a whole constellation of healthy choices that together result in a healthy lifestyle.

Heart Attack

Heart attack, or **acute myocardial infarction**, results from a sudden reduction in blood flow in the coronary arteries that supply the heart muscle, usually as a result of atherosclerosis. Heart muscle tissue dies during a heart attack. It is a medical emergency and can lead to **cardiac arrest**. Heart attack can occur at any age.

FACTS ABOUT HEART ATTACK

- About 150,000 people a year in the United States die from heart attacks. Many could have been saved by prompt care.

- Heart attack results from coronary artery disease, which often can be prevented or minimized with a healthy diet, exercise, not smoking, control of blood pressure and regular medical care.

- Heart attack is more likely in people with a family history of heart attacks.

- One-fifth of heart attack victims do not have chest pain – but often have other symptoms.

Signs and Symptoms of Heart Attack

The signs and symptoms of heart attack vary considerably, from vague chest discomfort (which the victim may confuse with heartburn) to crushing pain, with or without other symptoms. The victim may have no signs and symptoms at all before collapsing suddenly. Sometimes the victim has milder symptoms that come and go for two or three days before the heart attack occurs.

It is important to consider the possibility of heart attack with a wide range of symptoms rather than expecting a clearly defined situation, including a lack of chest pain or discomfort.

Note that some heart attack symptoms are more common in women. Chest pain or discomfort is still the most common symptom, but women are somewhat more likely to have shortness of breath, jaw or back pain, indigestion, and nausea and vomiting. Common signs and symptoms include:

- Complaints of persistent discomfort, pressure, tightness, ache or pain in the chest
- Pain may spread to neck, shoulders or arms
- Shortness of breath
- Feelings of indigestion
- Dizziness, lightheadedness or feeling of impending doom
- Pale, moist skin or heavy sweating
- Patients often deny symptoms

Care for Heart Attack

It is important to act quickly when a victim may be having a heart attack, because death from heart attack usually occurs within an hour or two after symptoms begin. Care for a heart attack victim begins with calling for help. In an out-of-hospital setting, call 9-1-1 to get help on the way immediately as well as an AED if one is not already at the scene. Then help the victim rest in the most comfortable position. A sitting position is often easiest for breathing. Loosen any constricting clothing. Try to calm the victim, and reassure him or her that help is on the way. Do not let the victim eat or drink anything. Because heart attack frequently leads to cardiac arrest, be prepared to give BLS if needed. Administer supplemental oxygen to the victim if it is available and you are trained in its use (Appendix B). Ask the victim if he or she is taking heart medication; if so, help obtain the medication for the victim. Follow the directions on the medication.

In recent years the value of aspirin as a clot-preventing medication has become well known, and many health care providers advise their patients who are at risk for cardiovascular disease to take one low-dose aspirin daily unless they are allergic or experience side effects such as gastrointestinal bleeding. Unless the victim is allergic or cannot take aspirin for any other reason, encourage the victim to chew one uncoated adult aspirin or two low-dose baby aspirin.

Nitroglycerin is often of benefit to a heart attack victim who already has this prescription drug. Nitroglycerin increases blood flow through partially restricted arteries by dilating them. Nitroglycerin is generally prescribed for angina, a condition of pain in the chest caused by narrowed coronary arteries. If the victim has nitroglycerin, you can assist him or her in using it. Nitroglycerin comes in small tablets that are dissolved under the tongue, tablets that dissolve in the cheek, extended release capsules, oral sprays and extended-release patches that are applied to the chest – usually daily **(Figure 3-2)**. Follow the victim's instructions to help with the drug. Do not attempt to give the drug yourself if the victim is unresponsive.

Angina

Angina pectoris, usually just called angina, is chest pain caused by heart disease and usually occurs after intense activity or exertion. Other factors may trigger the pain of angina, such as stress or exposure to extreme heat or cold. The pain is a sign that the heart muscle is not getting as much oxygen as needed, usually because of narrowed or constricted coronary arteries. The pain usually lasts only a few minutes, during which time the person should rest. The pain may also radiate to the jaw, neck, or left arm or shoulder. People usually know when they have angina and may carry medication for it, usually nitroglycerin.

If the victim identifies the symptoms as those of angina, help the person take his or her own medication and rest. If the pain persists more than 10 minutes or stops and then returns, or if the victim has other heart attack symptoms not relieved by rest, give care as for a heart attack.

Cardiac Arrest

Cardiac arrest may be caused by:

- Heart attack or other heart disease
- Drowning
- Suffocation
- Stroke
- Allergic reaction
- Diabetic emergency
- Prolonged seizures
- Drug overdose
- Electric shock
- Certain injuries
- Any condition causing respiratory arrest

CPR is needed for all victims in cardiac arrest. You do not need to know the cause of cardiac arrest before starting CPR.

Cardiopulmonary Resuscitation (CPR)

CPR helps keep the victim alive by circulating some oxygenated blood to vital organs. Compressions on the **sternum** (breastbone) increase pressure inside the chest, resulting in movement of some oxygen-carrying blood to the brain and other tissues. Rescue breaths move oxygen into the lungs, where it is picked up by the blood. The circulation of blood resulting from CPR is not nearly as strong as the circulation from a heartbeat, but it can help keep the brain and other tissues alive until a normal heart rhythm is restored. Often an electric shock from an AED (see Chapter 4) or other medical procedures called **advanced cardiac life support (ACLS)** are needed to restore a heartbeat – and CPR can keep the victim viable until then. In some instances, the heart may start again spontaneously with CPR.

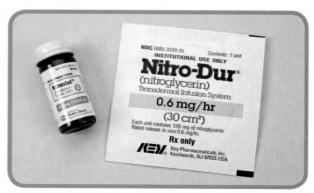

Figure 3-2 *Nitroglycerin tablets and patch.*

CPR has been demonstrated to save lives in many circumstances. With the most common cause of cardiac arrest, a heart attack, CPR and defibrillation within 3 to 5 minutes after the victim collapses can save more than 50% of victims. Given that sudden cardiac arrest occurs in more than 900 people with heart disease every day, CPR and use of an AED could save many thousands of lives every year. Remember that CPR is only one step in the cardiac chain of survival, however: in most cases of cardiac arrest, CPR only helps keep the victim alive until an AED and/or EMS professionals arrive at the scene.

Chest Compressions in CPR

The general technique of CPR involves alternating chest compressions and rescue breaths. After the initial assessment and determining the victim is not breathing normally and has no pulse definitely felt within 10 seconds, start CPR with chest compressions followed by rescue breaths. For a victim of any age, these are the general steps of CPR:

1. Bare the chest and find the correct hand position on the lower half of the breastbone in the middle of the chest in adults and children **(Figure 3-3)**. In infants, the position is just below the nipple line. For adults, place the heel of one hand in the correct position; then put the second hand on top of the first and interlock fingers. For children, depending on their size and your strength, use both hands or the heel of one hand. For infants, use two fingers.

2. Compress the chest hard and fast at a rate of at least 100 compressions per minute. Compressions in an adult should be at least 2 inches deep. In an infant or child, compressions should be at least ⅓ the depth of the chest (about 1½ inches in an infant or about 2 inches

in a child). Between compressions let the chest return to its normal height by taking your weight off your hands, but do not remove your hands or fingers from the chest.

3. If you are alone, alternate 30 chest compressions and 2 rescue breaths for all victims. In two-rescuer CPR for an infant or child, alternate 15 compressions and 2 breaths. For all victims, give each breath over 1 second.

Note: If supplemental oxygen equipment is present and you are trained in its use, give the victim oxygen during CPR (see Appendix B).

Rescue Breaths in CPR

Rescue breathing, once called mouth-to-mouth resuscitation, is a technique for blowing air or oxygen into a non-breathing person's lungs to oxygenate the blood. If the victim has no pulse, rescue breaths are combined with chest compressions in CPR to help circulate the oxygenated blood to vital organs.

Rescue breaths are given with the rescuer's own exhaled air unless special equipment is available. The air around us contains about 21% oxygen, and the breath we exhale is about 16% oxygen – still enough oxygen to increase the oxygen level in the victim's blood to maintain life.

Rescue breathing involves several important considerations, including opening the victim's airway before giving a breath, using a barrier device to reduce the risk of infection and using the technique correctly. These are discussed in the sections that follow.

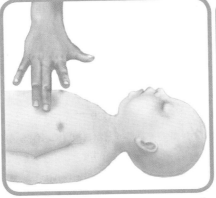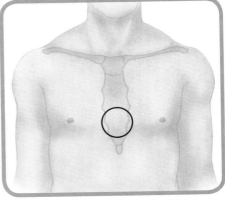

Figure 3-3 *Hand placement for chest compressions in CPR.*

Opening the Airway

The airway is the route by which air moves from the mouth and nose through the throat (pharynx) and into the lungs. The airway may be blocked by something stuck in the throat, by swollen airway tissues in a victim with a severe allergic reaction or a neck injury, or by an unresponsive victim's own tongue. The tongue can block the airway in an unresponsive victim lying on the back because of the weight of the tongue and relaxation of the muscles.

In an unresponsive victim, you need to ensure the airway is open before giving rescue breaths. When the victim is lying face up, you must prevent the tongue from obstructing the airway by positioning the victim's head to open the airway. The technique used to open the airway depends on whether the victim may have a spinal injury.

In a victim not suspected of having a spinal injury, tilt the head back and lift the chin as shown in **Figure 3-4**. This is called the head tilt–chin lift. This position moves the tongue away from the opening into the throat to allow air to pass through the airway **(Figure 3-5)**.

If the victim may have a spinal injury, do not tilt the head back to open the airway. Instead, lift only the jaw upward using both hands **(Figure 3-6)**. This is called a jaw thrust. The jaw thrust technique can be difficult to use, particularly when positioning a face mask. If you cannot successfully open the airway with the jaw thrust, however, then switch to the head tilt–chin lift method. It is more important to

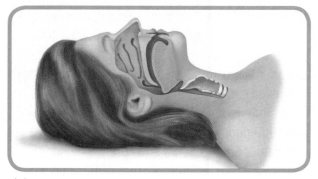

(a)

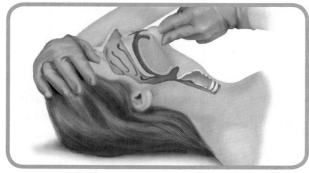

(b)

Figure 3-5 *(a) In an unresponsive victim, the tongue may block the airway. (b) The head tilt–chin lift opens the airway.*

open the airway than to be overly concerned with a possible spinal injury.

Giving Rescue Breaths

After opening the airway, give two breaths. Using a barrier device to prevent infection, such as a pocket face mask, or sealing your mouth over the victim's mouth, blow air into the victim over 1 second. Watch for a rise and fall in the victim's chest to ensure your breath is entering the victim's lungs. If your first breath does not go in, attempt to reposition the victim with the head tilt–chin lift or jaw thrust to ensure the airway is open, and try again. If your next breath still does not go in, the victim is choking. Give care as described in Chapter 5.

Use of Barrier Devices

Barrier devices are always recommended when giving rescue breathing. Two common types of barrier devices are pocket masks and face shields **(Figure 3-7)**. Both devices offer protection from the victim's saliva and other fluids, as well as

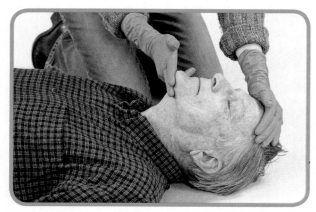

Figure 3-4 *Head tilt–chin lift.*

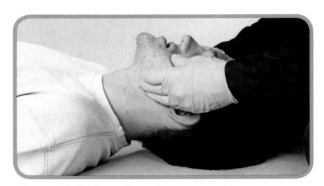

Figure 3-6 *Jaw thrust.*

from the victim's exhaled air when the barrier is equipped with a one-way valve. With either device, keep the victim's head positioned to maintain an open airway as you deliver rescue breaths through the device.

Face Mask

The **resuscitation mask**, often called a pocket face mask or simply a face mask, seals over the victim's mouth and nose and has a port through which the rescuer blows to give rescue breaths. A one-way valve allows the rescuer's air in through the mouthpiece, while the victim's exhaled air exits the mask through a different opening.

When using a face mask, it is essential to seal the mask well to the victim's face while maintaining an open airway. How you hold the mask depends on your position by the victim, whether the head tilt–chin lift or jaw thrust technique is used to open the airway, and whether you have one or two hands free to seal the mask. The following hand positions assume you have both hands free to seal the mask, whether alone at the victim's side while performing CPR or at the victim's head while another rescuer provides chest compressions.

From a position at the victim's side (solo rescuer giving CPR) using the head tilt–chin lift:

1. With the thumb and index finger of your hand closer to the top of the victim's head, seal the top and sides of the mask to the victim's head as shown in **Figure 3-8a**.

2. Put the thumb of your second hand on the lower edge of the mask.

3. Put the remaining fingers of your second hand under the jaw to lift the chin.

4. Press the mask down firmly to make a seal as you perform a head tilt–chin lift to open the airway.

From a position at the top of the victim's head (two rescuers giving CPR, or single rescuer performing rescue breathing without CPR) using the head tilt–chin lift:

1. Put your thumbs and index fingers on both sides of the mask as shown in **Figure 3-8b**.

2. Put the remaining fingers of both hands under the angles of the victim's jaw on both sides.

3. As you tilt the head back, press the mask down firmly to make a seal as you lift the chin with your fingers.

From a position at the top of the victim's head using the jaw thrust:

1. Without tilting the victim's head back, position your thumbs on the mask the same as for the head tilt–chin lift from the top of the victim's head, with fingers under the angles of the jaw.

2. Lift the jaw to open the airway as you press down with your thumbs to seal the mask, without tilting the head back **(Figure 3-8c)**.

Face Shield

Like a mask, a face shield is positioned over the victim's mouth as a protective barrier. The victim's nose, however, must be pinched closed when giving a rescue breath to prevent the air from coming out the nose instead of entering the lungs.

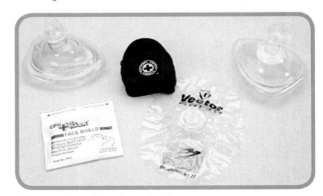

Figure 3-7 *Barrier devices.*

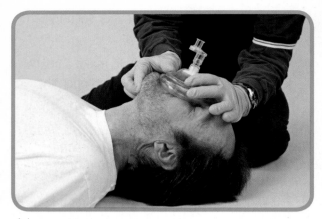

(a)

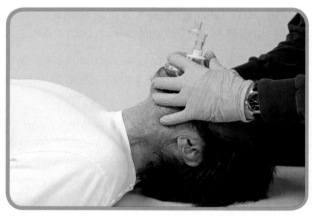

(b)

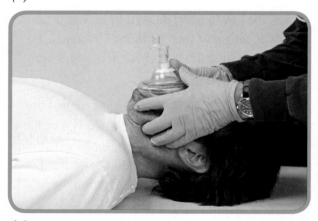

(c)

Figure 3-8 *(a) Face-mask hand position with rescuer at victim's side. (b) Face-mask hand position with rescuer at victim's head using the head tilt–chin lift. (c) Face-mask hand position used with jaw thrust for a victim with spinal injury.*

Bag Mask

Bag mask (or bag-valve-mask, or BVM) units, like regular face masks, protect the rescuer from disease transmission, but they are also more effective for providing ventilations and give non-breathing victims a greater concentration of oxygen. Appendix B describes how to use a BVM.

If No Barrier Device Is Available

If no barrier device is available, give rescue breathing directly from your mouth to the victim's mouth, nose or stoma if present. The risk of disease transmission is still very low.

Mouth to Mouth

Pinch the victim's nose shut and seal your mouth over the victim's mouth. Blow into the victim's mouth, watching the chest rise to confirm that the air is going in, and then remove your mouth to let the air escape.

Mouth to Nose

If the victim's mouth cannot be opened or is injured, or if you cannot get a good seal with your mouth over the victim's mouth, give rescue breathing through the nose. Hold the victim's mouth closed, seal your mouth over the nose to blow in and then allow the mouth to open to let the air escape.

Mouth to Stoma

Because of past illness or injury, some people breathe through a hole in their lower neck called a **stoma**. To give rescue breaths, cup your hand over the victim's nose and mouth to prevent your air from coming out the nose and mouth instead of entering the lungs. Then seal your mouth or barrier device over the stoma, and give rescue breaths as usual. A round pediatric face mask may produce a better seal around the stoma than a standard face mask.

Mouth to Nose and Mouth

Because of their smaller size, infants and very small children are generally given rescue breathing through both their mouth and nose. Seal your mouth over both the nose and mouth and give gentle breaths as usual, watching to see the chest rise with each breath.

Technique for Rescue Breaths

With the victim on his or her back, open the airway using the head tilt–chin lift, or the jaw thrust if the victim may have a spinal injury. Use a barrier device but do not delay rescue breathing to get one. The basic technique of rescue breathing is to blow air into the victim while watching the chest rise to make sure your air is going into the lungs. Do not try to rush the air in or blow too forcefully. Do not take a big breath in order to exhale more air into the victim; just take a normal breath. Give each breath over about 1 second. If the breath does not go in, if you feel resistance or do not see the victim's chest rise, then try again to open the airway. If your breath still does not go in, then the victim has an airway obstruction and needs care for choking (see Chapter 5).

Rescue Breaths for Infants

Rescue breathing for infants is similar to that for adults and children, with these differences:

- Gently tilt the head back to open the airway – do not overextend the neck.

- If no barrier device is available, cover both mouth and nose with your mouth to give breaths. (If you cannot cover both, use either the mouth or nose.)

Special Circumstances for Rescue Breaths

In some circumstances you may have to adjust how you give rescue breaths, including a victim vomiting, a victim wearing dentures, and a victim with facial injuries.

Vomiting

Usually, if the head is positioned correctly to open the airway and rescue breaths are not given too forcefully or too fast, the air will move through the trachea into the lungs rather than down the esophagus to the stomach. In some cases, however, air may move into the stomach. If the airway is not sufficiently open, if rescue breaths are given too quickly or if you continue to blow in air even after the lungs have expanded and the chest has risen, air may be forced into the stomach, making vomiting more likely. Vomiting presents two problems. If an unresponsive victim vomits, you have to roll the victim onto the side to drain the mouth, and then wipe the mouth clean before continuing rescue breathing. Vomiting also increases the risk of **aspiration**. Although a victim may vomit even with correct rescue breaths, to help prevent vomiting:

- Open the airway before giving a breath.

- Watch the chest rise as you give each breath.

- Blow steadily over 1 second.

- Stop each breath when the chest rises, rather than continuing to blow.

- Let the chest fall between breaths.

Dentures

A victim's dentures are usually left in place during rescue breathing. If they are loose and make it difficult to give breaths or may fall back in the mouth and block the airway, remove dentures before giving rescue breaths.

Facial Injuries

If the victim's mouth cannot be opened or is injured, or if you cannot get a good seal with your mouth over the victim's mouth, you can give rescue breathing through the nose. Hold the victim's mouth closed, seal your mouth over the nose to blow in and then allow the mouth to open to let the air escape.

Note: A victim with injuries may have blood in the mouth, which needs to be drained before giving rescue breathing. If suction equipment is available and you are trained in its use, you may suction either blood or vomit from the victim's mouth (see Appendix B).

Single-Rescuer CPR for Adults and Children

See "Skill: CPR for Adults and Children (1 Rescuer)" for the steps for combining chest compressions with rescue breaths in CPR for adults and children.

Skill CPR for Adults, Children and Infants (1 Rescuer)

1 Determine that the victim is not breathing normally and has no pulse. Activate the emergency response system.

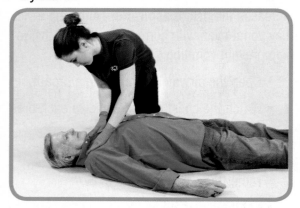

2 Expose the chest. Put your hand on the breastbone in the middle of the chest for chest compressions. For an adult, put your second hand on top of the first and interlock the fingers. For a child, use 1 or both hands. For an infant, put your 2 middle fingers of one hand just below the nipple line.

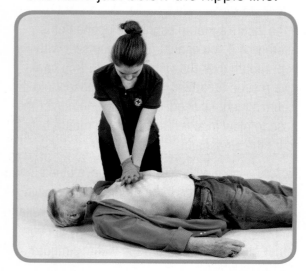

3 Give 30 chest compressions hard and fast at least 2 inches deep in an adult and at least ⅓ the depth of the chest in an infant (about 1½ inches) or child (about 2 inches) at a rate of at least 100 per minute. Count aloud for a steady fast rate: "One, two, three . . ."

4 Open the airway and give 2 rescue breaths, each lasting 1 second, to cause a visible chest rise. (If the first breath does not go in, reposition the victim's head and try again; if the second breath still does not go in, give choking care (see Chapter 5).

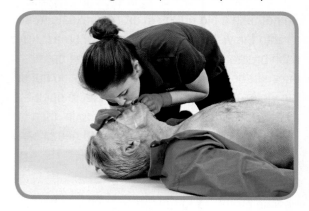

5 Continue cycles of 30 compressions and 2 breaths.

6 Continue CPR until:
- The victim is breathing normally and has a pulse.
- An AED is brought to the scene and is ready to use.
- Personnel with more training arrive and take over.

7 a. If the victim starts breathing normally and has a pulse but is unresponsive, put the victim in the recovery position and monitor breathing and pulse.

b. When an AED arrives, start the AED sequence for a victim who is not breathing normally and has no pulse.

ALERT

Chest Compressions

- Be careful with your hand position for chest compressions. Keep fingers off the chest.
- Do not give compressions over the bottom tip of the breastbone.
- When compressing, keep your elbows straight and keep your hands in contact with the chest at all times.
- Remember to compress the chest hard and fast but let it recoil completely between compressions.
- Minimize the amount of time used giving rescue breaths between sets of compressions.
- Performing chest compressions only is called Hands-Only CPR. It can be used by any bystander to treat adult victims of out-of-hospital cardiac arrest.

Two-Rescuer CPR for Adults and Children

When two rescuers at the scene are trained in CPR, resuscitation performed by both offers several advantages. Two-rescuer CPR:

- Minimizes the time between rescue breaths and compressions, making CPR more effective
- Allows for more quickly setting up an AED
- Reduces rescuer fatigue

The first rescuer begins by checking the victim for responsiveness and breathing. If the victim is not breathing normally, this rescuer checks for a pulse. Meanwhile, the second rescuer ensures 9-1-1 has been called and an AED is on the way, and moves into position on the opposite side of the victim to give chest compressions if the victim does not have a pulse. After 30 compressions, the first rescuer gives 2 rescue breaths, and CPR continues.

Two-rescuer CPR is performed in the same cycles of 30 compressions and 2 breaths for an adult (15 compressions and 2 breaths for an infant or child). One rescuer gives the chest compressions at a rate of at least 100 compressions per minute, and the other rescuer gives 2 rescue breaths. The rescuer giving compressions should count aloud during the compressions and pause after the last compression to let the other rescuer give 2 breaths. See Skill: CPR for Adult or Child (2 Rescuers).

The rescuers should switch positions about every 2 minutes (about 5 cycles of 30 compressions and 2 breaths) to prevent ineffective compressions resulting from fatigue. This change should be done at the end of a full CPR cycle after breaths are given, and should be accomplished in less than 5 seconds. It is recommended that positions be switched during any intervention that interrupts compressions (such as when the AED delivers a shock).

If an AED is present at the scene, the first rescuer gives both chest compressions and breaths while the second rescuer sets up the unit and attaches the pads (see Chapter 4). Then the rescuers resume CPR together.

Note: You may be assisting a professional with a higher level of training who places an advanced airway in the victim for ventilation. With an advanced airway in place, chest compressions are given continually at a rate of at least 100 per minute without pauses for rescue breaths. Ventilations are provided with a ventilation bag every 6 to 8 seconds (8 to 10 breaths per minute) while compressions are ongoing.

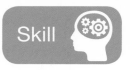

Skill · CPR for Adult or Child (2 Rescuers)

1 At the victim's head, Rescuer 1 checks for unresponsiveness and normal breathing. If the victim is not breathing normally, he checks for a pulse for no longer than 10 seconds. Rescuer 2 ensures that an AED has been summoned. At the victim's side, Rescuer 2 locates the site for chest compressions.

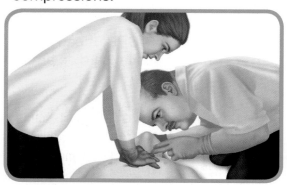

2 Rescuer 1 indicates, "No pulse." Rescuer 2 gives 30 compressions for an adult (15 for a child) at rate of at least 100 per minute, counting aloud for a fast, steady rate, then pauses.

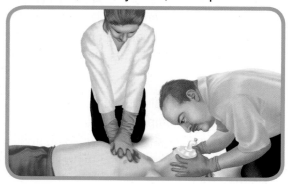

3 Rescuer 1 gives 2 breaths.

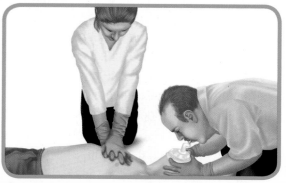

4 Rescuers continue cycles of 30 compressions in an adult (15 in a child) and 2 breaths for about 2 minutes (or after 5 cycles of compressions and ventilations at a ratio of 30:2) before switching compressor and ventilator roles. The switch should be done quickly (in less than 5 seconds).

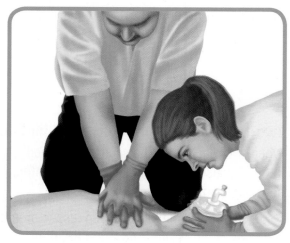

5 Rescuers continue CPR until:
- The victim is breathing normally and has a pulse
- An AED is brought to the scene and is ready to use
- Help arrives and takes over

6 a. If the victim starts breathing normally and has a pulse but is unresponsive, put the victim in the recovery position and monitor breathing and pulse.

b. When an AED arrives, start the AED sequence for a victim who is not breathing normally and has no pulse.

Transitioning from One-Rescuer CPR to Two-Rescuer CPR

In some situations a rescuer is already giving CPR when a second rescuer arrives on the scene. The rescuers should coordinate their actions for a smooth transition from one-rescuer CPR to two-rescuer CPR. The second rescuer moves into position on the other side of the victim to prepare to take over chest compressions. The first rescuer completes a series of compressions. While the first rescuer then gives 2 breaths, the second rescuer takes the correct hand position and begins compressions immediately after the second breath. For the next 2 minutes, the new rescuer gives chest compressions and the first rescuer gives rescue breaths.

Note: If you are the first rescuer who started CPR, the arriving second rescuer may be a rescuer with a higher level of training. In such a case, this rescuer assumes authority for how CPR should best be continued. If this rescuer determines your breathing or compression technique is inadequate, he or she may ask you to take on the other role — or may take over the CPR alone.

Two-Rescuer CPR for Infant

Two-rescuer CPR for an infant uses a different hand position for chest compressions from single-rescuer CPR. The rescuer giving compressions places the thumbs of both hands together in the correct position on the infant's sternum (just below the nipple line). The fingers of both hands encircle the infant's chest (**Figure 3-9**). The chest is compressed with both thumbs, as described in "Skill: CPR for Infant (2 Rescuers)". If you cannot encircle the infant's chest (e.g., the infant's chest is too large or the rescuer's hands are too small), use the single-rescuer method of performing compressions with 2 fingers.

When Not to Perform CPR

Generally, BLS skills should be performed on any victim who is not breathing and has no pulse. Exceptions in which it is acceptable to not give CPR to a victim include these:

- A Do Not Resuscitate order is present.
- The victim is obviously dead (decapitation, incineration or clear signs of prolonged death such as rigor mortis).
- It is not safe to be on the scene and the victim cannot be moved somewhere safe.
- A physician pronounces the victim dead.

Respiratory Emergencies

Any illness or injury that results in a victim no longer breathing, or breathing so ineffectively that the body is not receiving sufficient oxygen, even when a pulse is present, is a respiratory emergency. The two primary types of breathing emergencies are respiratory distress. A respiratory emergency can result from many different causes, such as:

- A physical obstruction in the airway, such as food blocking the pharynx or immersion in water
- An injury to the chest
- An illness affecting the lungs or airway, such as emphysema or asthma
- Heart problems
- An electrical shock
- A drug overdose or poisoning
- A severe allergic reaction

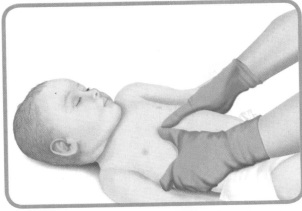

Figure 3-9 *The chest-encircling hand position for infant chest compressions when two professional rescuers are giving CPR.*

(continues on page 33)

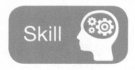

Skill CPR for Infant (2 Rescuers)

1 At the infant's head, Rescuer 1 checks for normal breathing and a pulse. At the infant's feet, Rescuer 2 positions hands in the chest-encircling position for chest compressions with both thumbs.

2 If pulse is absent, Rescuer 1 says, "No pulse." Rescuer 2 gives 15 chest compressions at a rate of at least 100 per minute, counting aloud for a fast, steady rate, then pauses.

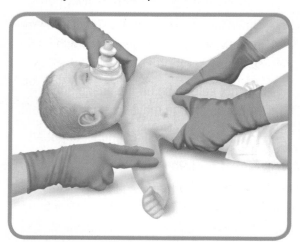

3 Rescuer 1 gives 2 breaths.

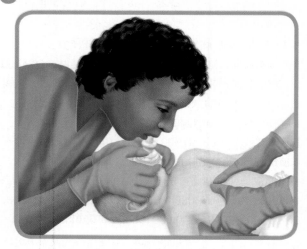

4 Rescuers continue cycles of 15 compressions and 2 breaths for about 2 minutes before switching compressor and ventilator roles. The switch should be done quickly (in less than 5 seconds). Rescuers continue CPR until:

- The infant is breathing normally and has a pulse.
- More advanced help arrives and takes over.

5 a. If the infant starts breathing normally but is unresponsive, hold the infant in the recovery position and monitor breathing and pulse.

b. When an AED arrives, start the AED sequence for an infant who is not breathing normally and has no pulse.

(continued from page 31)

Regardless of the cause, body cells begin to die soon after losing their oxygen supply. Brain cells are very susceptible to low levels of oxygen and begin to die as soon as 4 minutes after oxygen is cut off. Within 6 minutes, brain damage is likely. Death is likely soon after.

Respiratory arrest means breathing has completely stopped. With **respiratory distress**, the victim is still breathing, but the breathing may be difficult and becoming a serious problem. **Inadequate breathing** may also occur in an unresponsive victim who is breathing so slowly that oxygen levels in the blood are dropping to life-threatening levels.

Respiratory Distress

A victim in respiratory distress may be gasping for air, panting, breathing faster or slower than normal, or making wheezing or other sounds with breathing. Typically the victim cannot speak a full sentence without pausing to breathe. The victim's skin may look pale or ashen and be cool and moist; the lips and nail beds may be bluish. Lowered oxygen levels in the blood may make the victim feel dizzy or disoriented. The victim may be sitting and leaning forward, hands on knees, in what is called the tripod position.

Because respiratory distress in an infant or child may rapidly progress to arrest, it is crucial to act quickly when an infant or child has a problem breathing. In addition to the signs and symptoms described before, an infant or child may have flaring nostrils and more obvious movements of chest muscles with the effort to breathe.

Call for help immediately for any victim with sudden unexplained breathing problems. Help the victim rest in position of easiest breathing (often sitting up). Ask the victim about any prescribed medicine he or she may have, and help the victim take it if needed. For example, an asthmatic victim may need help using a **bronchodilator**, or a victim of a severe allergic reaction might need help with an emergency epinephrine auto-injector such as

an **EpiPen** **(Figure 3-10)**. Stay with the victim and be prepared to give BLS if the victim becomes unresponsive. Administer supplemental oxygen to the victim if it is available and you are trained in its use (see Appendix B).

Respiratory Arrest and Inadequate Breathing

Respiratory arrest and inadequate breathing are life-threatening emergencies. If an adult victim is breathing at a rate less than 10 breaths per minute, take this as a sign of inadequate breathing – the victim is not receiving sufficient oxygen. While many children will become bradycardic (an abnormally slow heart rate) when in respiratory arrest, an infant or child may have a pulse of 60 or higher per minute but still be breathing inadequately. In a victim who is not breathing adequately, do not wait for respiratory arrest before beginning to provide rescue breaths.

For a victim with an adequate pulse, rescue breathing is used by itself without chest compressions. Rescue breaths are given at a rate of one breath every 5 to 6 seconds (or every 6-8 seconds if an advanced airway is in place) in an adult; every 3 to 5 seconds for a child; or every 3 seconds for an infant. "Skill: Rescue Breathing" describes the sequence of steps in rescue breathing.

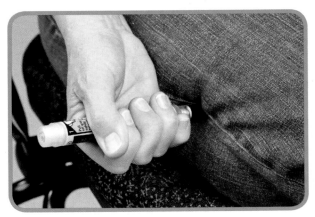

Figure 3-10 *Position the EpiPen firmly against the thigh to make the injection for anaphylaxis.*

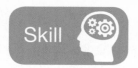

Skill **Rescue Breathing**

1 If the victim has a pulse but is not breathing normally, open the airway and give a breath over 1 second, watching the chest rise and letting it fall.

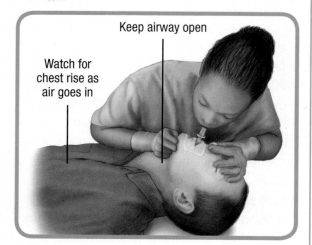

Keep airway open

Watch for chest rise as air goes in

2 If the first breath does not go in, try again to open the airway and give another rescue breath. If a breath still does not go in, the victim may be choking. Proceed to CPR for choking.

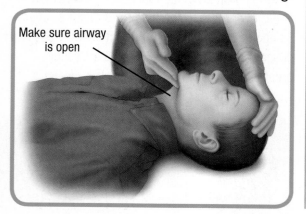

Make sure airway is open

3 If your breath goes in, continue rescue breathing. Give each breath over 1 second, at rate of 10 to 12 breaths per minute (1 breath every 5 to 6 seconds) for an adult; 12 to 20 breaths per minute for a child (1 breath every 3 to 5 seconds); or 20 breaths per minute for an infant (1 breath every 3 seconds).

4 Check the pulse about every 2 minutes. If there is no pulse, provide CPR beginning with chest compressions.

ALERT
- Do not blow harder than is needed to make the chest rise.
- After each breath, remember to let the air escape and the chest fall.
- Blowing in too forcefully or for too long is ineffective and may put air in the stomach, which may cause vomiting.

Compressions for Bradycardia in Infant or Child

In some circumstances, an infant or child may have a pulse but still have inadequate **perfusion** when being given rescue breaths or oxygen. If the pulse is less than 60 beats per minute and the infant or child has signs of poor systemic perfusion (such as poor skin color), provide CPR beginning with chest compressions. Do not wait for the victim to become pulseless if perfusion is poor even with ventilation with or without supplemental oxygen.

PREVENTING BREATHING EMERGENCIES

The common causes of respiratory arrest can often be prevented. They include choking (Chapter 5), drowning, and **sudden infant death syndrome (SIDS)**. In infants and children, most cardiac arrests follow respiratory arrest caused by choking.

Preventing Drowning

More than 3,000 people in the United States die each year from drowning. About two-thirds of these are adults and about a third are children under age 14. Approximately 6,000 additional near-drowning victims receive emergency treatment, and many of these will have permanent disabilities resulting from brain damage caused by lack of oxygen during submersion or related factors.

Drowning is the second leading cause of injury-related death for children 1 to 14 years old. Ninety percent of these drownings occur with an adult "supervising" but who is typically distracted by other factors. Attentive supervision is the best prevention, including watching infants in bathtubs or near buckets or toilets. Never leave a young child alone in or near a swimming pool, even if the child has had beginning swimming lessons or promises to stay out of the water in your absence. Protective barriers and locked gates also are important.

Half the drowning deaths among adolescents and adults are associated with alcohol use during recreational water activities. Prevention is simple: Don't drink and go into or near the water. Swim with a buddy, never dive into shallow or unknown water, and wear a personal flotation device (PFD) during water sports.

About 70% of the more than 500 annual boating deaths result from drowning. Most victims are not wearing a PFD, and about 40% of cases involve alcohol. Following safe boating guidelines would prevent most of these drowning deaths.

Preventing SIDS

Sudden infant death syndrome (SIDS), the sudden death of an infant younger than 1 of unexplained causes, occurs most commonly between 2 and 4 months of age. SIDS is the most common cause of infant death after 1 month of age. About 2,300 infants die of SIDS in the United States every year. It has been estimated that as many as 900 of the deaths attributed to SIDS each year may have resulted from simple suffocation, because these infants are found in suffocating environments and positions, often lying on the stomach with nose and mouth covered by soft bedding. To reduce the risk of SIDS and suffocation, always place infants on their back to sleep. Use a firm, flat crib mattress and remove pillows, comforters, toys and other soft objects from the crib. Do not cover the infant's head during sleep. Use only a thin blanket, and tuck it under the edges of the mattress at chest level and below. Avoid smoking – the risk of SIDS is much higher in infants exposed to passive smoke. Avoid overheating during sleep; dress the infant in light sleep clothing and keep the room at a temperature that is comfortable for an adult. Give an infant between 1 and 12 months of age a clean, dry pacifier at bedtime.

Conclusion

Remember that as important as CPR is for sustaining life, in many cases of cardiac arrest the victim also needs defibrillation to restore a normal heartbeat. Use of an AED is described in the following chapter. CPR is also used for unresponsive victims with an airway obstruction, as described in Chapter 5.

Review Questions

1. Vomiting during CPR may result from –
   a. blowing air in too forcefully.
   b. not blowing in enough air.
   c. compressing the chest too quickly.
   d. compressing the chest too deeply.

2. How long should it take to deliver one rescue breath?
   a. ½ second
   b. 1 second
   c. 1½ seconds
   d. 2 seconds

3. To open the airway of an unresponsive victim without suspected spinal injury –
   a. tilt the head back and lift the chin.
   b. thrust the jaw upward with both hands.
   c. tilt the head back while prying open the mouth.
   d. do not tilt the head back, but hold the chin down.

4. What is the correct position for the rescuer's elbows when giving CPR to an adult?
   a. Bent and locked.
   b. Straight and locked.
   c. Bent and flexible.
   d. Straight and flexible.

5. The common signs and symptoms of heart attack include –
   a. chest pain, fever and flushed skin.
   b. chest pain, headache and inability to raise both arms.
   c. chest pain, sweating and shortness of breath.
   d. chest pain, difficulty speaking or swallowing, and vision problems.

6. Which statement is true about the ratio of compressions and breaths when adult CPR is performed by two rescuers?
   a. Rescue breaths are given by one rescuer without the other rescuer pausing in chest compressions.
   b. A ratio of 15 compressions and 2 breaths is used for adults.
   c. A ratio of 5 compressions and 1 breath is used for adults.
   d. The usual ratio of 30 compressions and 2 breaths is used for adults.

7. The correct hand position for chest compressions in adults is –

    a. on the top of the breastbone below the neck.

    b. on the lower end of the breastbone just above the abdomen.

    c. on the lower half of the breastbone in the middle of the chest.

    d. three finger-widths above where the ribs join.

8. The preferred position for chest compressions in an infant when two health care providers are providing CPR is –

    a. two fingers just below the nipple line.

    b. both thumbs together just below the nipple, with fingers away from chest.

    c. both thumbs together just below the nipple line with fingers encircling the chest.

    d. both thumbs just below the nipple line, with about 2 inches separating the thumbs and the fingers encircling the chest.

9. The rate for rescue breathing for an adult victim who has a pulse but is not breathing is –

    a. 8 to 10 breaths per minute.

    b. 10 to 12 breaths per minute.

    c. 12 to 16 breaths per minute.

    d. 12 to 20 breaths per minute.

10. If you cannot successfully open a victim's airway with the jaw thrust –

    a. keep trying the jaw thrust with different head positions.

    b. tilt the head back but do not lift the chin.

    c. lift the chin but do not tilt the head back.

    d. use the head tilt–chin lift.

Case Scenario

As you step out of your vehicle at the scene to which you have been called, you see a group of people standing around a woman on the ground. As you approach, one person tells you he was the first one there; he found the woman motionless on the ground but has no idea what happened. You quickly perform the initial assessment and find she is not breathing and has no pulse. You are alone and do not carry an AED in your vehicle, but an ambulance has already been dispatched.

While positioning the woman on her back, you ask if anyone knows if there is an AED nearby, and someone rushes off to a nearby building to get one.

1. What should you do first?
   a. Give rescue breathing until the AED is brought to the scene.
   b. Call the 9-1-1 dispatcher back and ask for instructions.
   c. Start CPR, beginning with chest compressions.
   d. Put her in the recovery position.

2. CPR for this woman should consist of:
   a. Cycles of 15 compressions and 2 breaths, with compressions 1 to 1½ inches deep.
   b. Cycles of 15 compressions and 2 breaths, with compressions at least 2 inches deep.
   c. Cycles of 30 compressions and 2 breaths, with compressions 1 to 1½ inches deep.
   d. Cycles of 30 compressions and 2 breaths, with compressions at least 2 inches deep.

You give five cycles of compressions and breaths. She still is not breathing normally. Neither the ambulance nor the AED is yet at the scene.

3. What should you do next?
   a. Continue with additional cycles of compressions and breaths.
   b. Check her pulse for 30 seconds.
   c. Stop and wait for the AED to arrive.
   d. Speed up the rate at which you are giving compressions.

A minute or two later another trained professional rescuer arrives at the scene. Neither the ambulance nor the AED has yet arrived. The other rescuer offers to help.

4. How should you transition to two-rescuer CPR?
   a. Stop CPR until the second rescuer is ready, then start anew with one giving rescue breaths and one giving compressions.
   b. Complete the current cycle of compressions; the second rescuer takes position for compressions while you give 2 rescue breaths.
   c. While you are continuing compressions, the second rescuer simultaneously begins to give rescue breaths.
   d. Any of the above is acceptable.

Chapter 4 • Automated External Defibrillators (AED)

Not every victim who receives basic life support will benefit from an automated external defibrillator (AED), but many do. In many cases of cardiac arrest, the victim's heart has an abnormal rhythm that does not circulate the blood, and this rhythm can often be corrected with a shock from the AED. Remember the cardiac chain of survival: an AED should be used with any victim who is not breathing normally and has no pulse.

AEDS and Medical Direction

In many areas a health care provider oversees placement and use of the AED, and your AED training must meet certain requirements. For professional rescuers, this is called **medical direction**. Your course instructor will inform you how to meet the current requirements in your area for using an AED.

Laws regarding AEDs are changing. After the Food and Drug Administration approved nonprescription AEDs for home use in 2004, AED units that do not require specific training began appearing in homes and other settings. These devices have been demonstrated safe for use by lay people who follow the instructions printed on the device and given through sound prompts during use.

The Heart's Electrical System

The heart pumps blood to the lungs to pick up oxygen and pumps oxygenated blood to all parts of the body. The heart has four chambers: the left atrium, the right atrium, and the left and right ventricles. The ventricles, which are the lower chambers of the heart, do most of the pumping. The heart's electrical system keeps the four chambers of the heart synchronized and working together. The sinoatrial (SA) and atrioventricular (AV) nodes help organize and control the rhythmic electrical impulses that keep the heart beating properly **(Figure 4-1)**. The heart's normal rhythm is called the **sinus rhythm**.

With a heart attack or other heart problems, this rhythmic electrical control may be disrupted, causing an abnormal heart rhythm.

Ventricular Fibrillation

Ventricular fibrillation (V-fib) is the most common abnormal heart rhythm that occurs with cardiac arrest. Although we say a victim in V-fib is in cardiac arrest, the heart is not actually completely still but is beating abnormally. **Fibrillation** means the ventricles of the heart are quivering instead of beating rhythmically. Blood is not filling the ventricles and is not being pumped to the lungs or body as normal.

Heart attack is the most common cause of cardiac arrest and ventricular fibrillation is a common disrhythmia. Studies show that in approximately half the cases of cardiac arrest, the victim's heart is in fibrillation and therefore would benefit from a shock delivered by an AED.

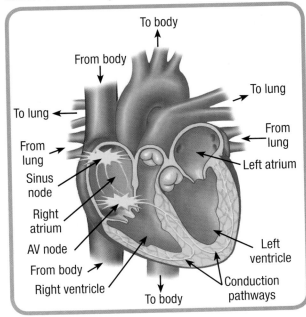

Figure 4-1 *The heart.*

How AEDs Work

The AED automatically checks the victim's heart rhythm by detecting electrical signals in the body picked up by the AED's **electrodes** (the pads). If the victim's heart is in V-fib, the AED will advise giving an electric shock in an attempt to return the heart to a normal rhythm. This is called **defibrillation**, or stopping the fibrillation of the heart **(Figure 4-2)**. The AED's electrodes, or pads, are placed on the victim's chest (or on the front and back of the chest, in a small child), and when the unit delivers a shock, electricity travels to the heart and "jolts" the heart's electrical system, often restoring a normal heartbeat.

Contemporary AEDs are easy and simple to use, but they must be used right away. Even when CPR is being given, with every minute that goes by before defibrillation begins, the victim's chances for survival drop by about 10%.

AEDs are complex inside but simple to use. They contain a battery or battery pack and are portable. All units have two pads connected to them with cables. These pads are placed on the victim's

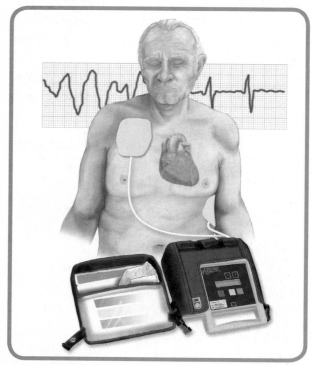

Figure 4-2 *An AED gives a shock to the heart.*

chest. The unit then analyzes the victim's heart rhythm and advises whether to give a shock. Some models have a screen that tells you what to do; all models give directions in a clear voice. AED models vary somewhat in other features, but all work in the same basic way **(Figure 4-3)**.

Using an AED

In any situation in which a victim suddenly collapses or is found unresponsive, be thinking about the possibility of cardiac arrest even as you come up to the victim. If someone else is present and you know an AED is available nearby, send that person to get it immediately. It is better to have it right away and not use it than to need it and have to wait for its arrival.

The steps for using an AED are simple:

1. Determine the need for an AED (no response, no normal breathing, no pulse).

2. Give CPR until the AED is set up and ready to use.

3. Attach the AED to the victim.

4. Allow the AED to analyze the victim's rhythm, and give a shock when the unit advises to shock.

AED and CPR

As always, first check the victim for responsiveness and normal breathing. If the victim is unresponsive and not breathing normally, call for help or send someone to call 9-1-1 and get an AED, before taking no more than 10 seconds to check for a pulse. Always use an AED if the victim is unresponsive, not breathing normally and has no pulse.

Use the AED on any unresponsive victim who is not breathing normally as soon as the unit is available. When two rescuers are present, one should give CPR while the other sets up the AED. Give 5 cycles of CPR (about 2 minutes) for a child found unresponsive and not breathing normally (not observed to have collapsed suddenly).

Attach the AED to Victim

Be sure the victim is not in water or in contact with metal. Water or metal conducts electricity that may pose a risk to you or others. Place the AED at the

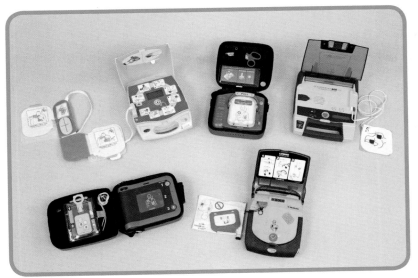

Figure 4-3 *A variety of AEDs.*

Analyze and Shock

With the pads in place and the AED unit on, most AED models then automatically analyze the victim's heart rhythm. Do not move or touch the victim while the unit is analyzing. After it analyzes the heart rhythm, the unit will advise you whether to give a shock or to resume CPR. If a shock is advised, be sure no one is touching the victim. Look up and down the victim and say, "Everybody clear!" Once everyone is clear, administer the shock (when advised) or stay clear as the AED automatically gives the shock. After the shock, immediately resume CPR, beginning with chest compressions, until the AED prompts to analyze the victim's heart rhythm again, usually after about 2 minutes. Then the AED will advise another shock if needed or prompt you to continue CPR (with the pads left in place).

Note that different AEDs may use different prompts. Follow the unit's voice and visual prompts through this process. Some units are programmed to administer the shock automatically rather than prompt the user to push the shock button; in this case, as always, follow the unit's prompts.

If the victim recovers (has a pulse and is breathing normally), put an unresponsive, breathing victim in the recovery position and continue to monitor breathing. Keep the AED pads in place, as some victims may return to V-fib and require defibrillation again.

The AED may also say no shock is indicated. This means the victim's heart will not benefit from defibrillation. If so, immediately continue CPR (see "Skill: Using an AED").

victim's side, next to the rescuer who will operate it. Turn it on, and attach the pads (electrodes) to the victim's chest. Most AED units have a diagram on the pads or the unit itself to remind you where to position the pads. Typically the first pad is placed on the right side below the collarbone and to the right of the breastbone. The second pad is placed below and to the left of the left nipple and above the lower rib margin. On an infant or small child, the AED unit may indicate to position the pads on the front and back of the chest instead. If you have only adult pads, use them on the infant or child because this is their only hope; position the pads on the front and back of the chest if they would be too close together on the anterior chest and possibly cause an electrical arc between them.

Attach the AED pads to the victim only if the victim is unresponsive and not breathing and there is no pulse. Expose the victim's chest, and dry the skin if needed with a towel or dry clothing (heart attack victims are often sweating). If the victim has heavy chest hair, quickly shave the pad areas. If a razor is not available, use scissors or trauma shears (which should be kept with the AED) to trim the hair and allow skin contact with the pads. Remove the backing from the pads and apply the pads firmly to the victim's chest. If required with your AED model, plug the pad cables into the main unit.

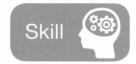
Skill **Using an AED**

1 Position the victim away from water and metal. Place the unit by the victim's shoulder and turn it on.

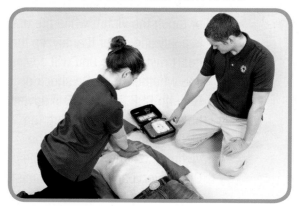

2 Expose the victim's chest, and quickly dry or shave the pad placement area if necessary.

3 Apply pads to the victim's chest as shown on pads. If needed, plug the cables into the unit.

Use adult pads for a victim 8 or older. For an infant or child younger than 8, use a unit with pediatric pads if available, applied as directed by the unit; if pediatric pads are unavailable, use adult pads.

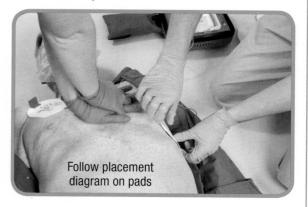

Follow placement diagram on pads

4 Stand clear during rhythm analysis.

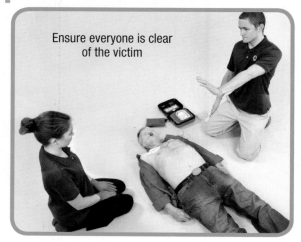

Ensure everyone is clear of the victim

5 Follow prompts from the AED unit to do one of three things: (1) press the shock button, (2) stay clear while the AED automatically delivers a shock or (3) do not shock but immediately give CPR with the pads remaining in place, starting with chest compressions.

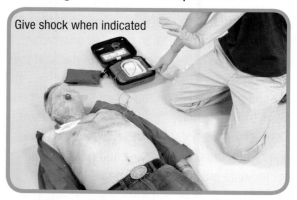

Give shock when indicated

6 Follow the AED's prompts to analyze the rhythm again after 5 cycles of CPR (about 2 minutes).

7 Continue steps 5 and 6 until the victim wakes up or more advanced help arrives and takes over.

8 If the victim begins breathing normally but is unresponsive, put the victim in the recovery position (with pads remaining in place) and continue to monitor breathing and pulse.

ALERT

- Move the victim away from metal or standing water before using the AED

- Remove any medication pads with a gloved hand, and dry the victim's chest well before attaching the electrodes.

- Avoid any flammable materials, including oxygen flowing through a mask. Do not use alcohol to wipe the victim's skin.

- Do not use the AED when in motion in a vehicle or boat.

- Do not use a cell phone or two-way radio within 6 feet of an AED.

- Remember not to touch the victim while the AED is analyzing the rhythm or administering a shock.

AEDs for Children and Infants

AEDs are now designed and recommended to be used for both children and infants. Follow the adult guidelines for children older than 8.

Although sudden cardiac arrest in younger children is much rarer, it can occur from causes such as:

- Sudden infant death syndrome

- Poisoning

- Drowning

- A heart problem

In most cases, however, cardiac arrest in a child is not caused by a heart problem, and in most cases the child's heart is not in V-fib. Therefore, give a child or infant 2 minutes of CPR before using the AED, unless the child or infant was witnessed to collapse suddenly. If the child does not recover, then use the AED as usual. This is different from the protocol for adults, in whom cardiac arrest is more likely to be the result of heart attack and on whom the AED should be used immediately.

Most AED units can be used with children and infants, using different pads specially designed for children and infants. It is important to use only approved pediatric AED electrode pads, which are smaller than those for adults and produce

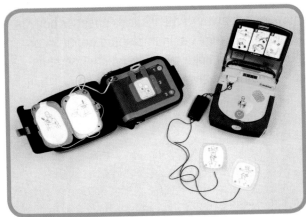

Figure 4-4 *The AED on the right has pediatric electrode pads. The one on the left uses a key to reduce the joules (electrical charge) to the adult pads for use with infants and children.*

lower-energy shocks, on a child younger than 8. Usually the pads have a distinctive appearance to prevent confusing adult and pediatric pads, such as pink connectors and teddy bear emblems. If pediatric pads are not available, using adult pads is better than not using the AED at all. Pediatric pads should not be used for an adult, however, because the lower energy is insufficient to affect the heart rhythm.

Be sure to follow the device's instructions for pad placement on a small child. For example, the

AED shown on the right in **Figure 4-4** uses pad placement on the front and back of the child's chest. Testing has demonstrated that with small children it can be difficult to position both the pads on the front of the chest, and studies have shown placement on the front and back also delivers an effective shock (see the box on page 46).

Special AED Considerations

Internal Pacemaker or Defibrillator

When you expose the victim's chest to apply the AED pads, you may see a bulge or lump beneath the victim's skin from an implanted **pacemaker** or defibrillator, often on the upper left side of the chest **(Figure 4-5)**. Do not place a pad directly over this area, but instead place it at least 1 or more inches away. If the victim's chest or body is jerking, there may be an implanted defibrillator that is giving shocks; wait until the jerking has ended before applying the pads.

Medication Patches

If the victim has a medication patch or paste on the chest, remove it with a gloved hand and wipe the chest before applying the AED pads **(Figure 4-6)**.

AED Problems and Maintenance

With regular maintenance, an AED should not have any problems during use. The AED may also prompt you to avoid problems. If you get a low-battery prompt, change the battery or battery pack before continuing. Another prompt may advise you to prevent moving the victim, if the AED detects motion. An error message may also appear if the electrodes are not firmly in contact with the victim's skin.

AEDs require regular maintenance. Check the manual from the manufacturer for periodic scheduled maintenance and testing of the unit. The battery or battery pack must be kept charged,

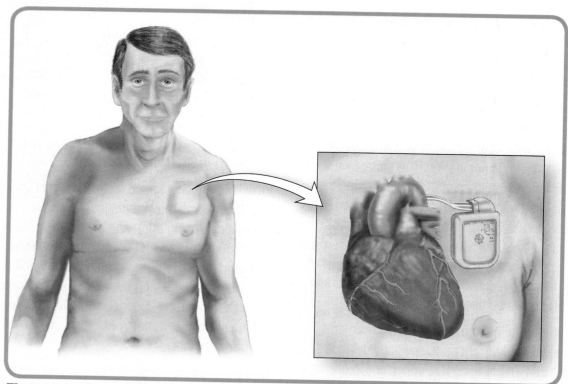

Figure 4-5 *Vary AED pad placement if there is an internal device.*

and a charged backup battery or battery pack should be available. Pads should be sealed and replaced on their expiration dates.

A daily inspection of the unit helps ensure the AED is always ready for use and all needed supplies are present. Professional rescuers usually inspect the unit at the beginning of their shift. Most facilities with an AED use a daily checklist form **(Figure 4-7)**. The checklist should always be adapted for the specific AED model, including the manufacturer's daily and periodic maintenance guidelines. In addition, many units come with a self-diagnostic test or simulator device to be used to check that the AED is correctly analyzing rhythms and delivering shocks; this may be part of the daily inspection routine.

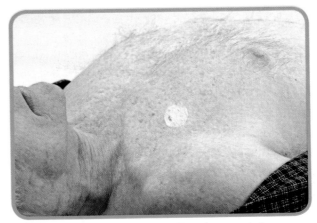

Figure 4-6 *Remove medication patches prior to AED pad placement.*

AED INSPECTION CHECKLIST

Date: _____ Location: _____ AED Model: _____

Inspected by: _____ Signed: _____

Criteria	ok/no	Corrective action/remarks
AED unit		
verify correctly placed	_____	_____
clean, clear of objects	_____	_____
no cracks or damage to case	_____	_____
cables/connectors present and not expired	_____	_____
fully charged battery in place	_____	_____
charged spare battery present	_____	_____
check status/service light indicator	_____	_____
check absence-of-service alarm	_____	_____
power on, self-test	_____	_____
Supplies		
Two sealed sets of electrode pads	_____	_____
Verify expiration date on pad packages	_____	_____
Razor	_____	_____
Medical exam gloves	_____	_____
Hand towels	_____	_____
Scissors or trauma shears	_____	_____
Pocket mask or face shield	_____	_____

Figure 4-7 *Example of an AED inspection checklist.*

CHANGING AED TECHNOLOGY

AEDs were first designed for use on adults and older children and therefore originally had pads that came in one size only and were placed in the typical manner on the upper right and lower left chest, as described earlier. When research showed the benefit of lower-energy shocks for pediatric victims, newer units were developed that used separate pediatric pads, sometimes placed on the front and back of the chest. AED technology continues to evolve, with some units able to determine characteristics of the victim and adjust the shock level automatically. Other new units now use the same pads for all victims, regardless of size and weight, but have a separate switch on the unit to use for pediatric victims. With such advances, separate pediatric pads may eventually become obsolete.

Conclusion

You have learned how rescue breathing, CPR and AED work together in the treatment of victims in cardiac arrest. These are crucial skills for professional rescuers, and they also require periodic refreshing to remain effective. Even if you are now becoming trained in CPR and AED, remember that to continue to use these lifesaving skills in the future, you will routinely need a refresher course.

Review Questions

1. Most AEDs administer a shock to the victim –
   a. whenever you turn it on.
   b. while you are giving rescue breaths during CPR.
   c. when you push the shock button after being prompted to do so.
   d. about 3 seconds after the pads are applied to the victim.

2. While the AED is giving the victim a shock, you should –
   a. continue CPR.
   b. not touch the victim.
   c. push the shock button repeatedly.
   d. push down on the pads to hold them in place.

3. An AED may be used on an infant or child if you –
   a. use pediatric pads.
   b. turn the voltage knob to a lower setting.
   c. put the pads on the arms to lower the voltage through the heart.
   d. put petroleum jelly between the skin and the pads.

4. The AED pads should be positioned where on the victim?
   a. Where the diagram on the unit or pads indicate placement.
   b. Below the nipples on both sides of the chest.
   c. In both armpits.
   d. One on the chest and the other on the abdomen.

5. If the AED indicates no shock is needed, you should then –
   a. wait 20 seconds and try again.
   b. remove the pads and turn the AED off.
   c. take the pads off and reposition them.
   d. give CPR starting with chest compressions.

Table 4-1: Summary of Basic Life Support

Step	Infant (under 1 year)	Child (1 – puberty, except 1 – 8 for AED)	Adult
1. Check victim for responsiveness and normal breathing.	Stimulate to check response. Observe whether breathing normally.	Tap shoulder and shout, "Are you OK?" while observing for normal breathing (gasps are not normal).	
2. If unresponsive, have someone call for help.	Send someone to call 9-1-1. If alone, give 2 minutes of care before calling 9-1-1 (and getting AED).	Send someone to call 9-1-1. If alone, unless the child has a known heart problem, give 2 minutes of care before calling 9-1-1 (and getting AED).	Send someone to call 9-1-1. If alone, call 9-1-1 and get an AED immediately (give 2 minutes of care first for drowning victim).
3. If unresponsive and not breathing normally, check pulse in less than 10 seconds.	Check brachial pulse.	Check carotid or femoral pulse.	Check carotid pulse.
4. If pulse is present but not normal breathing, start rescue breaths. Open airway.	Head tilt–chin lift (but do not overextend neck).	Head tilt–chin lift or jaw thrust.	
4a. Give 2 breaths.	Use barrier device or cover mouth, nose, or stoma. Each breath lasts 1 second.		
4b. If breaths go in and chest rises, continue rescue breathing.	1 breath every 3 seconds.	1 breath every 3-5 seconds.	1 breath every 5-6 seconds.
4c. If breaths do not go in, reposition head and try again.	Each breath lasts 1 second.		
4d. If breaths still do not go in, give care for airway obstruction.	Start CPR beginning with chest compressions. Check the mouth for an object each time breaths are given, and remove it if seen.		
5. If no pulse, give CPR, starting with chest compressions.	For compressions, use 2 fingers just below the nipple line. Compress chest to 1/3 the depth of chest, or about 1½ inches. (Two rescuers use 2-thumb-encircling hands technique.)	For compressions, use one or two hands in the center of the chest between nipples. Compress chest to 1/3 the depth of chest (about 2 inches).	For compressions use both hands, one on top of the other, in the center of the chest between nipples. Compress chest at least 2 inches.
5a. Chest compressions in CPR.	Chest compressions at a rate of at least 100 per minute.		
5b. Ratio of compressions and breaths – single rescuer.	Cycles of 30 compressions and 2 breaths.		
5c. Ratio of compressions and breaths – two rescuers.	Cycles of 15 compressions and 2 breaths.		Cycles of 30 compressions and 2 breaths. With an advanced airway in place, compressions are continuous and ventilations provided every 6 to 8 seconds.
6. If no pulse, use AED as soon as available.	Use pediatric electrode pads (or adult pads if pediatric pads are unavailable).		Use adult electrode pads.
7. If victim recovers normal breathing and pulse, put in recovery position.	Hold infant and monitor breathing.	Lay on side in HAINES recovery position and monitor breathing.	

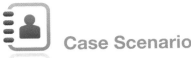

Case Scenario

You and your partner respond to a home where a man in his 40s has collapsed. Your partner is carrying the AED as you enter the house. The victim is on his side on the floor. His wife tells you he suddenly just passed out and fell to the floor.

1. What do you do first?
   a. Give him 2 rescue breaths.
   b. Check for responsiveness and normal breathing.
   c. Start CPR.
   d. Help your partner set up the AED.

You discover the victim is unresponsive and is not breathing. You quickly check for, but do not find, a pulse. Your partner is setting up the AED but it is not yet ready to use.

2. Now what should you do?
   a. Dry the victim's chest so he is ready for the AED pads.
   b. Give rescue breathing.
   c. Start CPR beginning with chest compressions.
   d. Put him in the recovery position.

Your partner has the AED ready and is applying the pads to the victim's chest. She tells you the unit is ready to analyze the victim's heart rhythm.

3. What should you be doing at this moment?
   a. Continue CPR until the unit completes its analysis.
   b. Ask your partner to assist you with CPR while the unit does the analysis.
   c. Give another 2 minutes of CPR before having the unit analyze the victim's rhythm.
   d. Do not touch the victim during the analysis.

The AED advises giving a shock. You stay clear of the victim, and your partner presses the button to administer a shock.

4. What is now your appropriate action?
   a. Take up to 30 seconds to check for a pulse.
   b. Continue CPR.
   c. Administer another shock.
   d. Put the victim in the recovery position.

After about 2 minutes of CPR, the AED analyzes the victim's rhythm again and does not advise a shock. You continue two-rescuer CPR with the pads still in place, and the victim moves and starts breathing. You check and find he has a pulse and is now breathing adequately. He remains unresponsive.

5. What do you do now?
   a. Remove the AED pads and keep the victim on his back with his head tilted to keep his airway open.
   b. Tell your partner to pack up the AED and return it to your vehicle while waiting for more help to arrive.
   c. Put the victim in the recovery position with the pads still in place, and monitor his breathing and pulse.
   d. Continue CPR.

4 • Automated External Defibrillators (AED)

Chapter 5 • Airway Obstructions

An airway obstruction is a life-threatening emergency because the victim is not getting oxygen. Basic life support includes skills to use for a responsive victim who is choking. CPR is used for unresponsive victims with an airway obstruction.

Airway Obstruction

A victim is said to be choking when the airway is obstructed either partially or fully. A victim can choke on:

- Food or other foreign bodies in the mouth

- The tongue (in an unresponsive victim lying on his or her back)

- Teeth or other body tissues resulting from injury

- Vomit

A complete **airway obstruction** means the victim is getting no air at all and consequently no oxygen is entering the blood. This victim will soon become unresponsive, and the heart will soon stop. Choking care is urgently needed: The airway must be cleared, and then rescue breathing or CPR must be provided as needed.

With a partial obstruction, the victim is still getting some air into the lungs. The victim may be able to cough out the obstructing object – or breathing may be very difficult, and the victim might be unable to cough strongly enough to expel the object.

Assessing Choking

Most cases of choking in adults occur while eating. Most cases of choking in infants and children occur while eating or playing. Often, therefore, someone is present and recognizes the choking event while the victim is still responsive.

Choking may be either mild or severe. With a mild obstruction the victim is usually coughing forcefully in an attempt to expel the object. The victim is getting some air and may be making wheezing or high-pitched sounds with breaths, along with coughing. Do not interrupt the person's coughing

or attempts to expel the object; do not pound the person on his or her back in an effort to help.

With severe choking, however, the victim is getting very little air or none at all. The person may look frantic and may be clutching at his or her throat. You may notice a pale or bluish coloring (cyanosis) around the mouth and nail beds. A victim who is coughing very weakly and silently, or not coughing at all, is unlikely to expel the obstructing object. The victim cannot speak. Ask the victim if he or she is choking. If the victim cannot answer but indicates that he or she is choking, ask for permission to help and begin choking care for a responsive victim. This is an urgent situation requiring immediate care.

An unresponsive victim who may be choking receives the same initial assessment as any unresponsive victim. If the victim is not breathing normally, check for a pulse in less than 10 seconds. Start CPR with chest compressions if no pulse is felt, or start rescue breathing if a pulse is present. If your first breath does not go into the victim after the airway has been opened, try again to open the airway and attempt a second breath. If it still does not go in, then assume that the victim has an obstructed airway.

Care for Choking Adults and Children

Choking care depends on whether the victim is responsive or unresponsive and whether, in a responsive victim, the obstruction is mild or severe:

- For a **responsive choking victim who is coughing**, encourage the coughing to clear the object. Stay with the victim and call 9-1-1 if the object is not immediately expelled.

- For a **responsive choking victim who cannot speak or cough forcefully**, give **abdominal thrusts** as described in "Skill: Choking Care for Responsive Adult or Child."

- For an **unresponsive victim who is not breathing normally and who may be choking**, immediately call (or have someone call) 9-1-1, and begin CPR.

With a responsive victim, after quickly asking for consent, telling the victim what you intend to do and having someone call 9-1-1, stand behind the victim and reach around his or her abdomen. Having one leg forward between the victim's legs helps you brace in case the victim becomes unresponsive and falls. Keep your head slightly to the side, in case the victim's head snaps back if he or she becomes unresponsive.

Make a fist with one hand, and place the thumb side of the fist against the victim's abdomen, just above the navel. Grasp the fist with your other hand and thrust inward and upward into the victim's abdomen with quick thrusts. The pressure of each thrust forces air from the lungs up the trachea to expel the object. Pause only briefly after each abdominal thrust to see if the victim is able to breathe or cough, and continue with additional thrusts if not.

If you are giving abdominal thrusts to a child or someone much shorter than you, kneel behind the victim. If the victim is much taller than you, ask the victim to kneel or sit, because it is important that your thrusts are upward as well as inward, which is impossible if you have to reach up to the victim's abdomen.

Note that because abdominal thrusts can sometimes cause internal injury, it is recommended that a victim who is treated with abdominal thrusts be examined by a medical professional.

When a severe obstruction is not cleared, the victim will become unresponsive within minutes. You may have found the victim in an unresponsive condition, or the victim may become unresponsive while you are giving abdominal thrusts if the object is not expelled. In the latter case, quickly and carefully lower the victim to lie on his or her back on the floor. Make sure 9-1-1 has been called. Begin the CPR sequence as usual with 30 chest compressions delivered hard and fast. Then when you open the victim's mouth to give rescue breaths, look first for an object in the mouth. If you see an object in the victim's mouth, remove it. If the object is expelled, give two rescue breaths as usual and continue CPR unless the victim recovers and is breathing normally.

If the obstruction remains, the chest compressions of CPR may expel the foreign object. While giving CPR, each time you open the victim's mouth to give breaths, check first to see if an object is visible, and remove it if it is. (See "Skill: Choking Care for Responsive Adult or Child and the Skill: Choking Care for Unresponsive Adult or Child.")

Care for Choking Infants

If a responsive choking infant can cry or cough, watch carefully to see if the object comes out. If the infant is responsive but cannot cry or cough, have someone call 9-1-1, and give the infant alternating back blows (slaps) and chest thrusts to attempt to expel the object. Support the infant in one hand against your thigh as you sit or stand, keeping the infant's head lower than the body. To prevent spinal injury, be sure to support the infant's head and neck during these maneuvers. The detailed steps for back blows (slaps) and chest thrusts are described in "Skill: Choking Care for Responsive Infant."

If an infant to whom you were giving responsive choking care then becomes unresponsive, send someone to call 9-1-1 (if this was not already done), and start CPR with chest compressions. As with an adult or child, the chest compressions may cause the object to be expelled. Check for an object in the mouth before you give a breath, and remove any object you see. Never do a finger sweep of the mouth if you do not see an object, as this could force an object deeper into the throat.

(continues on page 55)

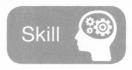

Skill — Choking Care for Responsive Adult or Child

1 Stand behind an adult victim with one leg forward between the victim's legs. Keep your head slightly to one side. For a child, move down to the child's level or kneel behind the child. Reach around the abdomen.

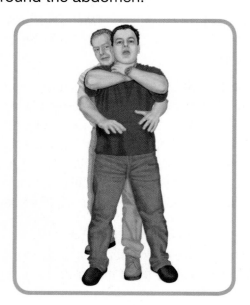

2 Locate the person's navel with a finger from one hand. Make a fist with the other hand and place the thumb side of the fist against the person's abdomen just above the navel.

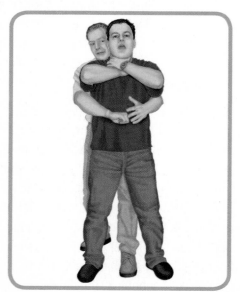

3 Grasp your fist with your other hand and thrust inward and upward into the victim's abdomen with quick thrusts. Continue abdominal thrusts until the victim expels the object or becomes unresponsive.

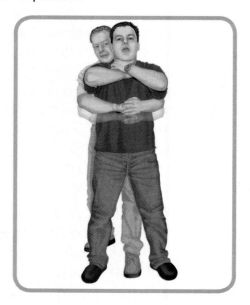

4 For a responsive pregnant victim, or any victim you cannot get your arms around or cannot effectively give abdominal thrusts to, give chest thrusts in the middle of the breastbone from behind the victim. Avoid squeezing the ribs with your arms.

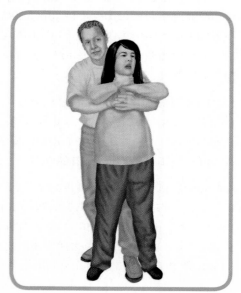

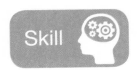
1 If the victim is unresponsive and not breathing normally, check for a pulse for no more than 10 seconds.

2 a. If no pulse, start CPR with 30 chest compressions at least 2 inches deep in an adult and at least 1/3 the depth of the chest in child (about 2 inches) at a rate of at least 100 per minute. Count aloud for a steady fast rate: "One, two, three, . . ."

    b. If the victim has a pulse, begin rescue breathing.

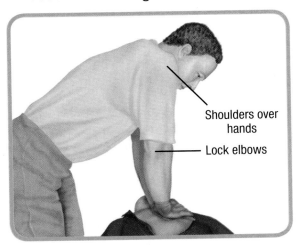

Shoulders over hands

Lock elbows

3 Open the airway with the head tilt–chin lift or jaw thrust.

4 Give two rescue breaths, each lasting 1 second. If the first breath does not go in and the chest does not rise, position the victim's head again to open the airway, and try again.

5 If breaths still do not go in, continue CPR with chest compressions, in a ratio of 30 compressions and 2 breaths.

6 Look inside the mouth before giving breaths after each cycle of compressions, and remove any object you see. Then give two breaths.

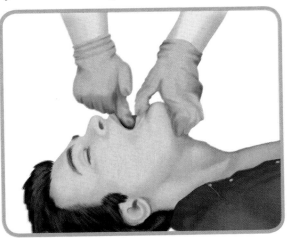

7 Continue CPR until:
- The victim recovers and is breathing normally.
- Additional help arrives and takes over.

5 • Airway Obstructions

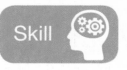

Skill · Choking Care for Responsive Infant

1 Support the infant face-down by holding the head in one hand, with the torso on your forearm against your thigh. Give up to 5 back blows (slaps) between the shoulder blades with the heel of your hand.

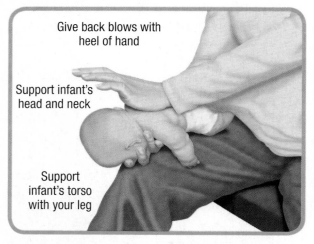

Give back blows with heel of hand

Support infant's head and neck

Support infant's torso with your leg

2 Check for an expelled object. If not present, continue with next step.

3 With your other hand on the back of the infant's head, roll the infant face-up, supporting the back of the infant's head with your hand.

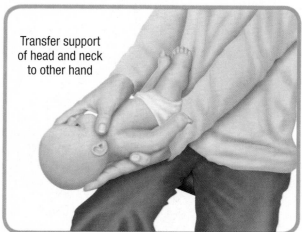

Transfer support of head and neck to other hand

4 Give up to 5 chest thrusts with two fingers on the sternum just below the nipple line, about 1 per second. Each thrust should be 1½ inches deep. Check mouth for an expelled object.

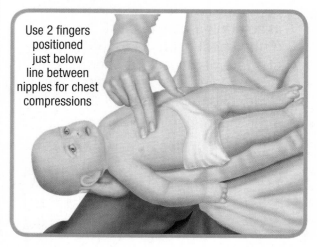

Use 2 fingers positioned just below line between nipples for chest compressions

5 Continue cycles of 5 back blows (slaps), 5 chest thrusts and checking the mouth. If alone, call 9-1-1 after 1 minute. Continue until the object is expelled or the infant becomes unresponsive. If the infant becomes unresponsive, give CPR. Look inside the mouth before giving breaths, after each cycle of compressions, and remove any object you see.

(continued from page 51)

When you encounter an unresponsive infant, first check for normal breathing. If the infant is not breathing normally, check quickly for a pulse and then begin CPR or rescue breathing. If your first breath does not go in after opening the airway and the infant's chest does not rise, try again after repositioning the infant's head to open the airway. If the second breath does not go in, assume that the infant has an airway obstruction and continue CPR, checking the mouth for an object each time you open it to give a rescue breath.

PREVENTING CHOKING

More than 4,000 people in the United States die from choking each year. Adults 65 and older are more than twice as likely to die from choking as younger adults, followed by young children.

In adults, choking often results from trying to swallow large pieces of food that have not been chewed sufficiently, eating too quickly or eating while engaged in other activities. Choking is more common in people under the influence of alcohol or drugs. Choking also is more likely in people wearing dentures, apparently because of a diminished ability to sense how well food has been chewed.

Choking is a serious threat to infants and children up to 3 or 4 years old, and a significant cause of death. An infant or young child may put any small object in his or her mouth, and nonfood items account for about 70% of choking deaths in infants and young children. Never leave small objects (such as buttons, beads or coins) within reach of an infant. Ensure that small parts cannot break off toys or other items around the infant or young child. Feed infants only soft foods that do not require chewing. Have children sit in a high chair or at a table to eat. Never let a child move around while eating. Teach children not to eat too fast or talk or laugh while eating. Cut into very small pieces any foods a child could choke on, such as hot dogs. Do not give children younger than 3 foods such as peanuts, popcorn, grapes or gum.

Conclusion

You have now learned the basic life support skills needed for victims with the most common threats to life. Remember always to approach the victim with the same initial assessment of responsiveness, normal breathing and pulse. Then give appropriate care including, as needed: rescue breathing, CPR and AED, and care for airway obstruction.

Review Questions

1. A victim with a severe airway obstruction –

   a. cannot speak or cough forcefully.

   b. cannot speak but can cough forcefully.

   c. can speak and cough weakly.

   d. can speak but only in short sentences.

2. If a victim can talk normally to you, he or she –

   a. does not have a life-threatening condition.

   b. does not have a spinal injury.

   c. does not have an airway obstruction.

   d. is not having a heart attack.

3. What increases the risk of choking in an adult?

   a. High blood pressure medication.

   b. Overcooked foods.

   c. Gum disease.

   d. Drinking alcohol with meals.

4. To give abdominal thrusts to a responsive choking adult, what hand position is used?

   a. Both hands together on the bottom edge of the breastbone.

   b. Both hands together just above the navel.

   c. One hand at the navel and one hand at the "V" where the lower ribs meet.

   d. One hand on the bottom rib at each side.

5. What is important when giving choking care to a responsive infant?

   a. Alternate series of back blows (slaps) and chest thrusts.

   b. Keep the infant's head raised above the body.

   c. Give CPR in the usual way.

   d. Perform a more gentle version of the adult responsive choking technique.

Case Scenario

You are at lunch in the company cafeteria. An employee has brought her 3-year-old son to work with her today, and they are seated not far from you. Suddenly the woman stands up, yelling for help. As you approach, you see the boy shaking his head frantically, clawing at his neck with both hands. His mother says he is choking. You identify yourself and ask if you can help.

1. What should you do first?
    a. Confirm that he is not breathing, move behind him and give abdominal thrusts.
    b. Position him on his back and start rescue breathing.
    c. Have him bend forward against one arm and pound on his back with your other hand.
    d. Give chest compressions the same as in CPR.

While you are providing care, the boy suddenly slumps forward, unresponsive. You lower him to the floor on his back.

2. Which of the following actions should you take first?
    a. Check his mouth for a foreign body.
    b. Start rescue breathing.
    c. Shout for someone to call for help.
    d. Give abdominal thrusts.

Another employee has called for more help.

3. What is the next step to take?
    a. Pound on his breastbone with the heel of one hand.
    b. Check his mouth again.
    c. Give CPR starting with chest compressions.
    d. Go get an AED.

Appendix A • Special Resuscitation Situations

Trauma

In most situations in which the victim is severely injured by blunt or penetrating trauma, problems with breathing or circulation are the result of the trauma rather than a coinciding problem. Do not assume, however, that a trauma victim has experienced only trauma, because another problem may have occurred first or at the same time. For example, a victim may have a heart attack and sudden cardiac arrest while on a ladder, resulting in a fall and possible fractures. A victim of drug overdose or poisoning may develop a severe breathing problem while operating machinery, causing an accident and traumatic injury. As a general rule, treat a trauma victim like any other: Perform the initial assessment and give basic life support as needed.

Trauma victims generally have a "call first" rather than "call fast" status. Trauma that is severe enough to cause cardiac arrest can only be helped by invasive procedures, usually in a hospital. If the victim is to have a chance of survival, advanced care must arrive as quickly as possible so a determination can be made about the next steps. The victim needs to be transported to definitive care as quickly as possible.

Depending on the nature of the trauma, the victim may have a spinal injury as well. Any blow to the body severe enough to impact breathing or circulation also is likely to potentially injure the spine. Remember to keep the head in line with the body when positioning the victim, and use the jaw thrust technique rather than head tilt–chin lift to open the airway.

Trauma to the head or face may result in blood or other fluid blocking the airway. Check the mouth when opening the airway, and if necessary wipe out any blood or vomit. With more extensive fluid, you may have to turn the victim onto one side to let it drain from the mouth. If the equipment is available and you are trained in its use, suction the victim's mouth when opening the airway (see Appendix B).

In cases of cardiac arrest in victims with severe trauma, local protocol may include not using the AED, as these victims usually do not have a heart rhythm that improves with the AED. Always follow your local protocol, and if the AED is not used, give CPR as usual while waiting for advanced help.

Hypothermia

Hypothermia is low core body temperature as a result of exposure to a cold environment, often by immersion in cold water. Hypothermia requires special consideration when providing emergency care. Severely cold temperatures make the victim susceptible to heart rhythm problems, but a thorough assessment is important because some of these victims have been successfully resuscitated after a long period of hypothermia or immersion.

In severe hypothermia, the victim's heart may be beating very slowly or may be in arrest, and the respiratory rate also may be very slow or have stopped. For an unresponsive victim who is not breathing normally, check for a pulse no longer than 10 seconds, and if a pulse is not definitely felt, start CPR immediately. Follow local protocol for use of an AED with a hypothermia victim.

Do not delay or stop resuscitation efforts to rewarm the victim, but if possible prevent further heat loss from the victim's body. Other rescuers can remove wet clothing, for example, or cover the victim with a blanket while basic life support is ongoing. Be gentle when handling or moving a hypothermia victim, because the heart is susceptible to dysrhythmias precipitated by motion or jarring.

Near Drowning

In any situation in which a victim is in the water, ensure your own safety before attempting a rescue. It is very dangerous for an untrained rescuer to enter the water to rescue a responsive victim, who may grab the rescuer and make rescue difficult or impossible. Reach to the victim with a pole or long object, throw a rope or floating object, or go to the victim in a watercraft if possible. Beginning rescue breaths as soon as possible is a high priority for drowning victims. If you can do so, begin rescue breaths (after confirming respiratory arrest) even before removing the victim from shallow water.

It is necessary to remove the victim from water, however, to give CPR. With an unresponsive victim removed from the water, consider whether the nature of the incident suggests a possible spinal injury, such as diving in shallow or murky water or being thrown against the shore in surf conditions. If the cause of the submersion is unknown, assume the victim may have a spinal injury. Keep the head in line with the body when moving or positioning the victim, and use the jaw thrust technique rather than a head tilt–chin lift to open the airway.

Begin the initial assessment as usual by checking for responsiveness. Remember that this is a "call fast" rather than "call first" situation. If you are alone, give care for about 2 minutes (rescue breathing or CPR) before stopping to go for help.

Note that BLS care for a drowning victim is somewhat different from that given other victims found unresponsive. A drowning victim is more likely to have a pulse and may need only rescue breathing without chest compressions. If the victim is not breathing normally, first open the airway and give two rescue breaths. Then quickly check for a pulse. If the victim has a pulse but is still not breathing normally, continue with rescue

breathing as described in Chapter 3. If the victim does not have a pulse, give CPR immediately, beginning with chest compressions.

Do not take any special actions to try to remove water from the victim first.

If the victim is not breathing and your rescue breaths do not make the chest rise, open the airway again and try to give 2 breaths. If your breaths still do not go in, give chest compressions for an airway obstruction.

If supplemental oxygen is available and you are trained in its use, administer oxygen to the victim (see Appendix B). When an AED is available and is ready to use, use it as usual. Victims have been resuscitated after being submerged in cold water for an extended time. If the victim may be hypothermic, follow the special considerations described earlier.

Electric Shock

Electric shock may result from a lightning strike or contact with a source of household current or high-voltage power lines. The shock may cause breathing to stop because of paralyzed respiratory muscles and may cause cardiac arrest by disrupting the heart's electrical controls.

Remember scene safety before approaching the victim. Downed power lines or household or industrial electrical appliances or cords may still be "live" and pose a threat to rescuers. Call 9-1-1 for downed power lines, and do not attempt to move them yourself or move the victim away from them. For electrical appliances, first shut the power off at the circuit breaker box or unplug the power cord if it is safe to do so.

Electric shock may cause a range of injuries in addition to effects on respiration and circulation. Especially with a high-voltage shock, such as that caused by lightning, the victim my have severe burns and possible fractures due to strong muscular contractions caused by the electrical shock. With a lightning strike victim, assume there may be spinal injury.

When it is safe to approach the victim, perform the initial assessment and provide care as needed. If the victim has a pulse but is not breathing, provide rescue breathing and continue to check the pulse. If the victim has no pulse, provide CPR and call for an AED. Often an electric shock causes ventricular fibrillation, in which case the AED may return the heart to a normal rhythm. If alone, first activate the emergency response system, get an AED if one is available, and then return to provide CPR.

Pregnancy

As described in Chapter 5, a woman in the late stages of pregnancy with an airway obstruction should be given chest thrusts rather than abdominal thrusts to expel an obstructing object. A responsive victim can be given chest thrusts from behind while standing, and an unresponsive victim is given chest thrusts in the same manner as the chest compressions of CPR. Note that chest compressions should be given slightly higher on the sternum of a pregnant woman.

When a pregnant woman at a gestational age beyond 20 weeks lies on her back, the enlarged uterus may press against the inferior vena cava, which returns blood to the heart from the lower half of the body. This pressure may decrease the blood flow to the heart and affect circulation to vital organs. When possible, therefore, position an injured pregnant woman lying on her left side, which reduces pressure from the uterus on the vena cava. Gently move the uterus to the left to help alleviate pressure.

When giving CPR to a pregnant woman at a gestational age beyond 20 weeks, if possible position her for chest compressions on a firm surface that can be tilted 27 degrees to 30 degrees such that her back is angled from the left lateral position (lying on left side).

Otherwise, perform basic life support skills on a pregnant woman in the same manner as other victims, including use of an AED in cases of cardiac arrest.

Appendix B • Advanced Resuscitation

In most emergency situations, professional rescuers can provide basic life support without specialized equipment or supplies beyond basic personal protective equipment such as gloves and a resuscitation mask. Several adjunctive devices, however, can enhance the effectiveness of resuscitation. These devices include suction devices to help keep the victim's airway clear, oral and nasal airways to help ensure air reaches the victim's lungs, bag mask units for more effective rescue breathing, and supplemental oxygen.

The resuscitation adjuncts you may use depend on both your training and your job description. Also, these devices may not be available in the emergency setting where you are caring for a victim. It is essential, therefore, to be able to perform BLS techniques such as rescue breathing and CPR without special equipment, as described in earlier chapters. In addition, resuscitative measures should never be delayed while waiting for adjunctive equipment.

When these devices are available and you are trained in their use, adjunctive devices increase the efficiency of resuscitation techniques and increase the victim's chances for full recovery.

Suction Devices

A **suction device** is used to clear blood, vomit and other substances from a victim's airway. These devices are generally safe and easy to use. Although different types of suction devices are available, they are similar in their use. Manual devices develop suction through a hand-pumping action, while other devices are powered by a battery or pressurized oxygen. Soft rubber bulb syringes are used for suctioning infants.

Suction devices for adults and children have a clear plastic tip that is inserted into the mouth or nostrils to suck out fluids and small solids. Different suction tips are available, varying from small, soft plastic tips that are more effective with fluids to larger, more rigid tips that are more effective for vomit and particulate matter. Some devices have a suction control port at the base of the tip that you cover with your finger to produce suction. As always, you should be familiar in advance with the specific equipment you may use in an emergency.

Suction is useful whenever a victim's airway may be obstructed – fully or in part – by body fluids, vomit or other matter. If the victim vomits when rescue breathing or CPR is underway, or if secretions or blood accumulate and impede ventilation, stop and quickly suction the mouth and/or nose and then continue resuscitation. An unresponsive breathing victim also may need suctioning to maintain an open airway. Usually you will know the airway needs suctioning when you hear gurgling sounds during breathing or ventilation.

The victim's head is turned to the side to help drain vomit or fluids before suctioning. If the victim may have a spinal injury, the victim must be turned on his or her side with the head and body in line as a unit, with the help of other rescuers. See "Skill: Suctioning (Adult or Child) and Skill: Suctioning (Infant)."

Safety precautions are necessary when suctioning. Because many suction devices generate strong suction pressures, be careful with the suction tip. Prolonged contact with mucous membranes in the mouth and nose can cause bruising, swelling and even bleeding. Never insert the suction tip farther than you can see. Prolonged suctioning also can decrease the volume of air reaching the victim's lungs. Vigorous suctioning may stimulate the victim's gag reflex, causing additional vomiting. Be especially careful not to suction too deep in an

(continues on page 64)

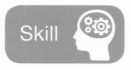

Skill Suctioning (Adult or Child)

1 Confirm that the suction device is working and produces suction.

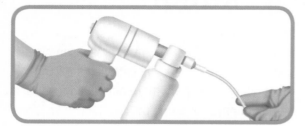

2 Turn the victim's head to one side and open the mouth (with spinal injury, support the head and turn with body as one unit).

3 Sweep out solids and larger amounts of fluid with your finger.

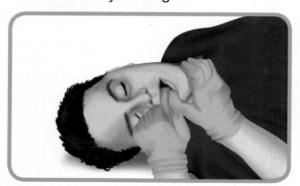

4 Determine the maximum depth of insertion by measuring the catheter tip from the earlobe to the corner of the mouth.

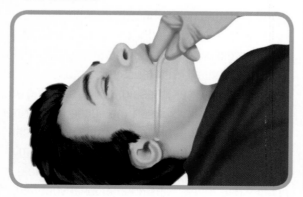

5 Turn on the suction, or pump the handle to create suction.

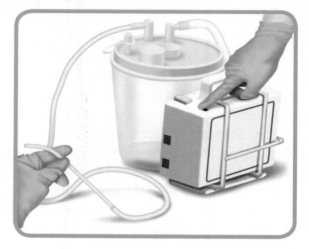

6 Insert the catheter tip carefully into the mouth. Put your finger over the proximal opening to begin suctioning, and move the tip about as you withdraw it.

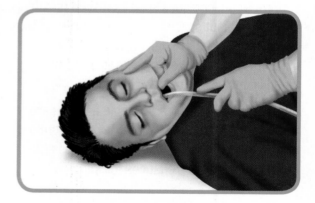

7 Reposition the victim's head with airway open, and begin or resume rescue breathing or CPR if needed.

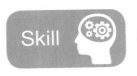

Skill Suctioning (Infant)

1 Hold the infant in position for suctioning, with the head lower than the body and turned to one side.

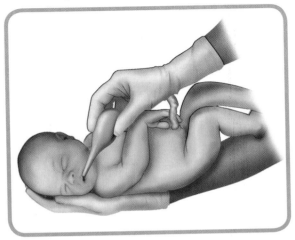

2 Squeeze the suction bulb first and then gently insert the tip into the infant's mouth.

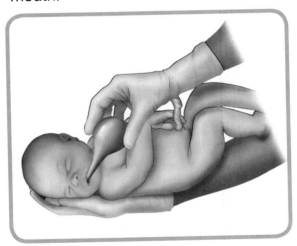

3 Gradually release the bulb to create suction as you withdraw the tip from the infant's mouth.

4 Move the bulb aside and squeeze it, with tip down, to empty it.

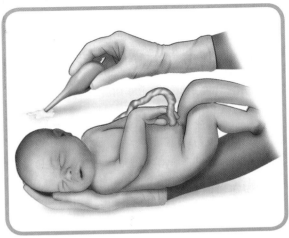

5 Repeat steps 2 through 4 until the airway seems clear, up to 3 times.

6 Repeat the suctioning steps for each nostril.

7 Begin or resume rescue breathing or CPR if needed.

B • Advanced Resuscitation

(continued from page 61)

infant. Always suction an infant's mouth before the nostrils, because suctioning the nose may stimulate the infant to breathe in and thereby inhale fluid or secretions from the mouth.

Remember standard precautions against disease transmission through body fluids. After the emergency, dispose of any contents in the reservoir of the suction device and clean the device according to the manufacturer's recommendations.

Airway Adjuncts

Oral and nasal airways are devices that help keep a victim's airway open during resuscitation or until the victim receives advanced medical attention. As discussed in Chapter 3, the most common cause of airway obstruction in unresponsive victims is the tongue. An airway device prevents this problem, and keeps the airway open more easily than head position alone while using resuscitation techniques or caring for a breathing victim. Supplemental oxygen can be given through a resuscitation mask or bag mask with an airway in place.

Oral Airways

Oral airways, also called **oropharyngeal airways**, are used only in unresponsive victims who do not have a gag reflex. If inserted into a responsive victim, or one who still has a gag reflex, the airway adjunct can cause vomiting. The victim's airway must be opened before the airway device is inserted; the device does not open the airway itself but will help keep it open. An oral airway can be used in an unresponsive victim who is breathing or who is receiving rescue breaths.

Proper placement of the oral airway is essential. An improperly placed airway device can compress the tongue into the back of the throat and further block the airway. Oral airways are curved so that they fit the natural contour of the mouth and are available in various sizes to ensure a proper fit **(Figure B-1)**. An airway adjunct that is too big can cause vomiting and may prevent the resuscitation mask from sealing well. An airway adjunct that is too small can slide into the back of the pharynx and

obstruct the airway **(Figure B-2)**. Remember to open the victim's airway before inserting the oral airway, as described in "Skill: Oral Airway Insertion." Periodically reassess the airway adjunct to confirm that it remains in proper position. A victim can be suctioned with an oral airway in place.

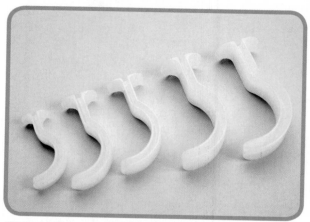

Figure B-1 - *Oral airways.*

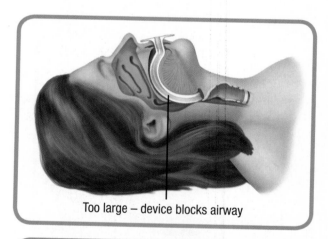

Too large – device blocks airway

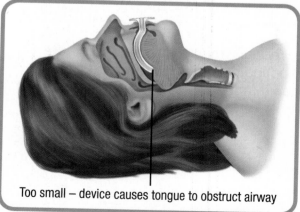

Too small – device causes tongue to obstruct airway

Figure B-2 *An oral airway that is too large or too small will obstruct the airway.*

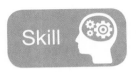
1 Choose an airway device of the correct size. (The oral airway length should match the distance from the corner of the mouth to the tip of the earlobe on the same side of the victim's face.)

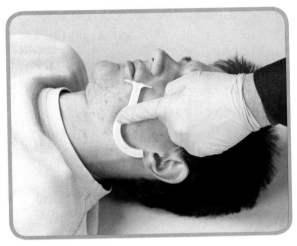

2 Open the victim's airway with a head tilt–chin lift or a jaw thrust, and open the mouth. Insert the airway device with the tip pointing toward the roof of the mouth.

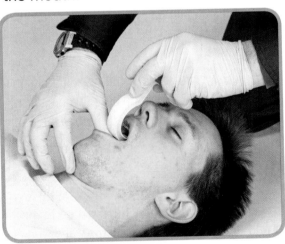

3 When the tip reaches the back of the mouth and you feel resistance, rotate the airway 180 degrees.

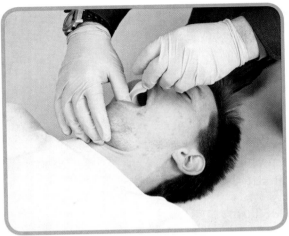

4 Continue to insert the airway device to its final position (with the flange resting on the lips).

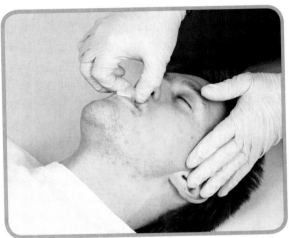

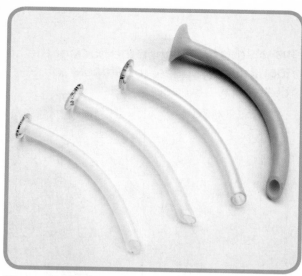

Figure B-3 *Nasal airways.*

Nasal Airways

A nasal airway, like an oral airway, helps maintain an open airway **(Figure B-3)**. A nasal airway (**nasopharyngeal airway**) can be used in a victim who is responsive or who, although unresponsive, has a gag reflex. Nasal airways also are effective for unresponsive victims with mouth or jaw injuries or tightly clenched teeth that prevent use of an oral airway. Nasal airways are less likely to cause gagging and vomiting than oral airways, but a disadvantage is that they are too narrow to suction through easily. Insert a nasal airway as described in "Skill: Nasal Airway Insertion," and continue to keep the victim's airway open with the head tilt–chin lift or jaw thrust. If needed, suction through a nasal airway using a small flexible suction catheter.

Resuscitation Masks and Bag Masks

Whether given by itself or as part of CPR, rescue breathing is performed more safely and effectively with a face mask. By using a mask, the rescuer avoids direct contact with the victim's mouth and thereby minimizes the risk of bloodborne and airborne disease transmission. The mask also makes it easier to ventilate the victim. The two primary types of masks used in emergencies are the resuscitation mask and the bag mask.

The resuscitation mask, often called a pocket face mask or simply a face mask, seals over the victim's mouth and nose and has a port through which the rescuer blows air to give rescue breaths. A one-way valve in the port allows the rescuer's air to enter through the mouthpiece while the victim's exhaled air exits the mask through a different opening. The rescuer's mouth is thereby protected from infection by the victim's air or body fluids. Chapter 3 describes how to seal a face mask to the victim's face and hold it in place. Face masks also have a port to which oxygen tubing can be connected so that supplemental oxygen can also be delivered through the mask. A face mask also can be used with an oral or nasal airway in place.

Bag mask (BVM) units also protect the rescuer but are more effective for providing ventilations to non-breathing victims because the victim receives air from the atmosphere (21% oxygen) rather than air the rescuer exhales (16% oxygen). The more oxygen delivered to the lungs, the more oxygen will reach the victim's vital organs to maintain life. Several different types of BVM units are available, but each has at least three components:

- The self-inflating bag holds the air or oxygen that is delivered to the victim when the bag is squeezed.

- The one-way valve allows air or oxygen to flow from the bag to the victim but prevents the victim's exhaled air from returning to the bag.

- The mask is similar to a resuscitation mask and is connected to the bag and valve; the proper size mask must be used for a proper fit.

An oxygen reservoir bag may be attached to the other end of the bag when supplemental oxygen is used **(Figure B-4)**.

To use the BVM on a non-breathing victim, position yourself above the victim's head. Perform a head tilt, and then position the mask on the victim's face. If you are alone, you need to hold the mask with one hand and squeeze the bag with the

(continues on page 68)

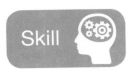
1 Choose the correct nasal airway size. (The nasal airway length should match the distance from the nostril to the tip of the earlobe on the same side of the victim's face.)

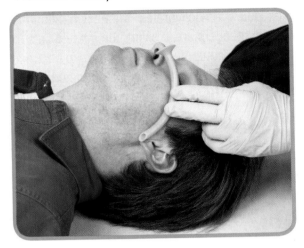

2 Coat the nasal airway with lubricant.

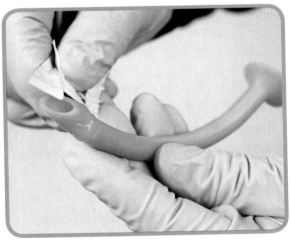

3 Insert the nasal airway in the right nostril with the bevel toward the septum.

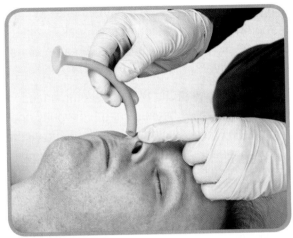

4 Insert the nasal airway straight back, sliding it along the floor of the nostril.

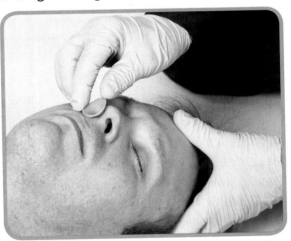

5 Insert the nasal airway until the flange rests against the nose.

B • Advanced Resuscitation

(continued from page 66)

other. To hold the mask in place with one hand, use the C-clamp technique, with thumb and index finger on the edges of the mask while the other fingers lift the jaw into the mask. If you are unable to open the airway and obtain a good seal with one hand, provide rescue breaths mouth to mask or mouth to mouth. A single rescuer skilled in its use may use a BVM when rescue breaths alone are being given.

Two-rescuer use of the BVM is recommended whenever possible because of the difficulty one person may have sealing the mask on the victim's face with one hand while squeezing the bag with the other. When a second rescuer is available to help with the BVM, one rescuer holds the mask in place using both hands while the second rescuer squeezes the bag, as shown in "Skill: Bag Mask (BVM) for Rescue Breathing (2 Rescuers)." Squeeze a 1-liter adult bag about ½ to ⅔ of its volume. Squeeze a 2-liter adult bag about ⅓ its volume. Squeeze the bag over 1 second, watching the victim's chest rise. Give a ventilation every 5 to 6 seconds in an adult (or every 3 to 5 seconds in a child, or every 3 seconds for an infant), the same as with rescue breathing by mouth or resuscitation mask.

When using a BVM, monitor the effectiveness of ventilations. Be careful to give rescue breaths at the usual rate and not hyperventilate the victim. Watch for the rise and fall of the victim's chest, and feel for resistance as you squeeze the bag. An increased resistance may mean blood or vomit is in the airway, or the airway is no longer open. A problem also can occur with sealing the mask to the victim's face, especially when a single rescuer must do this with one hand. If air is escaping around the mask, try repositioning the mask and your fingers. If you cannot obtain an adequate seal and the victim's chest does not rise with ventilations, or there are any other problems with using the BVM, use an alternate technique, such as a resuscitation mask, instead.

If available, supplemental oxygen should be used with the BVM (see the next section). An oxygen reservoir bag is attached to the valve on the bag, and the oxygen tubing attached to the bag. The device is used the same way to give ventilations, only now oxygen rather than air is being delivered to the victim. The reservoir holds oxygen being delivered to the device so the bag always fills with oxygen to be delivered in the next ventilation. When two rescuers are present, the second sets up the oxygen equipment and prepares to connect it to the BVM while the first begins providing rescue breathing with the BVM alone.

The BVM can be used with a non-breathing infant in the same manner as with an adult or child. Be sure to choose a mask of the correct size. Squeeze the bag only enough to make the chest rise, avoiding forceful squeezing or over-inflation that may lead to vomiting.

Supplemental Oxygen

In many emergency situations the victim will benefit from receiving supplemental oxygen, if available. Victims receiving basic life support are often receiving insufficient oxygen because of respiratory or cardiovascular problems. The air around us is about 21% oxygen, and the air we breathe out (and into a victim's lungs during rescue breathing) is about 16% oxygen. Depending on the supplemental **oxygen delivery device**, the victim can receive oxygen at concentrations up to 100%.

(continues on page 70)

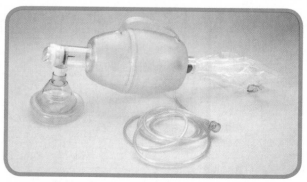

Figure B-4 *A single rescuer can use the BVM to provide rescue breathing, although use by two rescuers is recommended.*

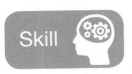
1 Rescuer 1 assembles the BVM with a mask of the correct size and puts the mask over the victim's mouth and nose.

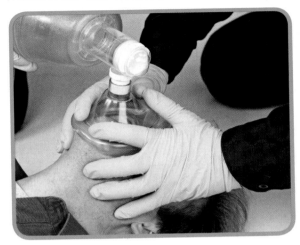

2 Rescuer 2 positions hands: thumbs and index fingers circling each side of the mask, the other three fingers of each hand behind the lower jawbone. Pull the jaw up into the mask instead of pushing the mask down on the jaw.

3 Rescuer 2 opens the airway and seals the mask to the victim's face.

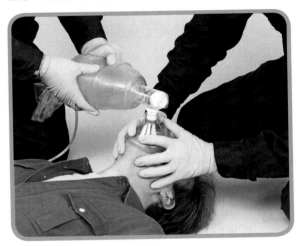

4 Rescuer 1 squeezes the bag to provide ventilations:

   a. 1 ventilation over 1 second in adult, every 5 to 6 seconds.

   b. 1 ventilation over 1 second in child, every 3 to 5 seconds.

   c. 1 ventilation over 1 second in infant, every 3 seconds.

5 Recheck pulse about every 2 minutes. If no pulse, call for an AED and start CPR.

B • Advanced Resuscitation

(continued from page 68)

Supplemental oxygen, when available, should be used along with other basic life support techniques, including rescue breathing and CPR. In addition, victims with serious medical conditions, including heart attack, stroke, seizures or serious injury, will potentially benefit from supplemental oxygen.

The following equipment is involved in giving supplemental oxygen:

- The oxygen source typically is a pressurized cylinder. When full, cylinders have a pressure of 2,000 pounds per square inch (psi). They come in various sizes and are usually painted green, although some stainless steel cylinders are not.

- The **pressure regulator** reduces the pressure of oxygen leaving the tank to a safe level and has a gauge that shows the pressure remaining within the cylinder. If the gauge reads 2,000 psi, the tank is full; if it reads 1,000 psi, it is half full; and so on. The pressure regulator is designed so that it works only with oxygen tanks.

- The **flowmeter**, used to adjust the rate of oxygen delivery, is usually built into the pressure regulator. The flow of oxygen reaching the victim is set by turning the calibrated flow valve.

- Oxygen tubing connects the cylinder to the delivery device. Connecting tubes are typically 4 to 5 feet long and have an adapter at each end.

- An oxygen delivery device, such as a face mask or **nasal cannula**, provides the flowing oxygen to the victim.

Safety Around Oxygen

Although oxygen itself does not burn, it vigorously supports combustion and creates a hazardous situation if used near an ignition source. Follow these guidelines around oxygen:

- Never allow smoking or an open flame near the oxygen source.

- Never use grease, oil or adhesive tape on the cylinder, pressure regulator or delivery device, because these are combustible.

- Never expose an oxygen cylinder to a temperature higher than 120° F.

- Never drop a cylinder or let it fall against another object. If the valve is dislodged, the cylinder can become a dangerous projectile powered by the compressed gas.

- Never try to use a non-oxygen regulator on an oxygen cylinder.

Oxygen Delivery Devices

Many different oxygen delivery devices are available, each with certain advantages and disadvantages. The following devices are most frequently used in emergency situations **(Figure B-5)**:

- Nasal cannulas, sometimes called nasal prongs, are used with breathing victims who do not require a high concentration of oxygen. The device has two small prongs that fit shallowly into the nostrils. The nasal cannula is easy to use and comfortable for the victim. The oxygen concentration delivered depends on the flow rate (1 to 6 liters per minute) and the victim's breathing rate, varying from about 24% to 50%.

- Resuscitation masks cover the mouth and nose and can be used for non-breathing victims receiving rescue breaths. Some masks have a special port for oxygen, which can be used for breathing victims who need oxygen. The mask then can be secured to the victim's head by an elastic band. A typical plastic face mask provides an oxygen concentration of 30% to 60% with a flow rate of 10 liters per minute.

- **Nonrebreathing masks** have a mask and a reservoir bag and are used with breathing victims. The oxygen fills the reservoir, which empties partially as the victim inhales. The victim's exhaled air escapes through a valve.

(continues on page 73)

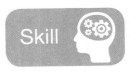
1 Check equipment: oxygen labels on the cylinder and regulator; tubing and delivery device ready.

2 Remove any protective seal, point the cylinder away, and open the main valve for 1 second.

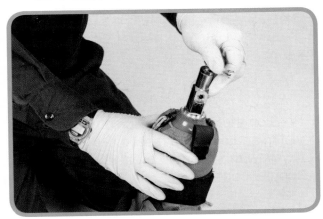

3 Remove any protective seals and attach the regulator to the oxygen cylinder.

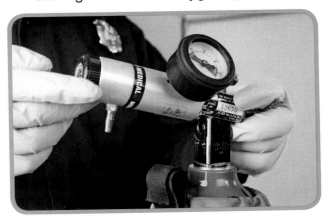

4 Open the main cylinder valve.

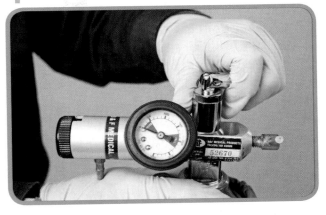

5 Check the pressure regulator gauge.

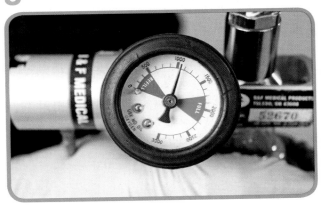

6 Attach the tubing to the flowmeter and the oxygen delivery device.

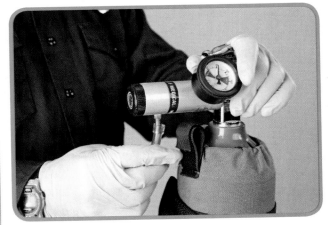

(continued)

B • Advanced Resuscitation

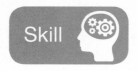
Skill **Oxygen Administration** *(continued)*

7 Set the flowmeter at the correct oxygen flow rate.
  a. 1–6 L/min for nasal cannula
  b. 10 L/min for face mask
  c. 10–15 L/min for BVM or nonrebreather mask

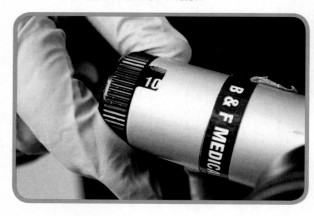

8 Confirm that the oxygen is flowing.

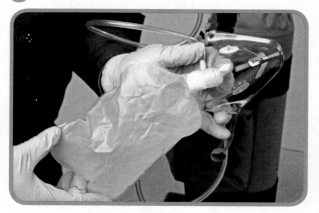

9 Position the delivery device on the victim and continue rescue breathing (or allow the victim to breathe spontaneously).

10 Monitor the pressure regulator gauge and be prepared to remove the delivery device and change tanks if the pressure drops below 500 psi. Observe oxygen safety precautions.

(continued from page 70)

With a minimum oxygen flow rate of 8 liters per minute, the oxygen concentration ranges from 80% to 95%. The flow rate is adjusted to prevent the reservoir from completely collapsing when the victim inhales. A firm mask fit is needed to prevent atmospheric air from entering the mask.

- Bag mask units, as described earlier, can also deliver oxygen either through a simple connecting tube to the bag or with an oxygen reservoir. Oxygen concentrations delivered to a non-breathing victim by a BVM with a reservoir can approach 100%. A BVM with a reservoir to receive oxygen also can be used for a breathing victim; unless the victim is having difficulty breathing, the bag is not squeezed.

Administration of Oxygen

"Skill: Oxygen Administration" describes the steps for setting up oxygen equipment and administering oxygen to the victim. Remember to follow safety principles when working with oxygen. If you are alone with a victim, do not stop providing basic life support to set up oxygen equipment. Give rescue breathing or CPR as needed, use the AED if present and appropriate, and care for other life-threatening problems first. Wait until the victim is relatively stable and breathing independently, or until another rescuer can help with the oxygen equipment. Once the victim is receiving oxygen, continue to monitor the flow of oxygen and tank pressure, as well as the victim's condition.

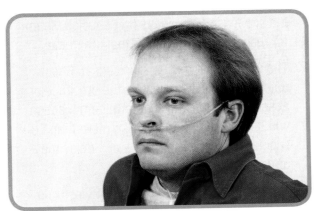

(a)

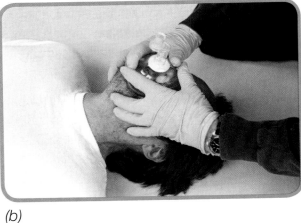

(b)

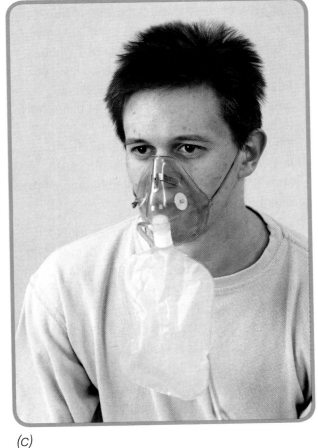

(c)

Figure B-5 *Oxygen delivery devices. (a) Nasal cannula. (b) Resuscitation mask. (c) Nonrebreathing mask.*

Appendix C • Answers to Review Questions and Case Scenarios

Chapter 1

Answers to Review Questions

1. d
2. b
3. a
4. c
5. c

Answers to Scenario

1. Answer choice d is the appropriate action to take. Victims who are not aware of the potential seriousness of their condition may at first refuse care but then accept it when they understand the possible consequences. Answer choices a and b put the victim at greater risk, and the victim has not definitively refused care because he has not yet learned the possible consequences of his actions. Answer choice c is inappropriate because Mark does not have the legal right to force the victim to accept care.

2. Answer choice a is correct: A professional rescuer must meet the standards of care (what one is trained to do). Because the victim is now unresponsive, Mark now has implied consent to give him lifesaving care such as CPR, and therefore he does not need consent from a family member. (This would also be a waste of valuable time in a life-threatening emergency.) Because this is a job responsibility, Mark does have a duty (legal obligation) to act.

Chapter 2

Answers to Review Questions

1. b
2. a
3. b
4. b
5. c

Answers to Scenario

1. The correct answer choice is b. After ensuring the scene is safe, always first check a victim for responsiveness and normal breathing.

2. The appropriate answer choice is d. Check quickly for a pulse, because the presence or absence of a pulse will determine the action you take next. But do not take more than 10 seconds to feel for a pulse – any delay may affect the victim's condition.

3. The correct answer choice is a. Always call for additional help – or have someone call. Even if you were alone in this situation, you would call as soon you recognized the victim was unresponsive and not breathing normally. It is critical to get an AED and advanced care on the way as soon as possible.

4. The appropriate answer choice is a. The victim is not breathing and has no circulation, and therefore needs CPR. You will use the AED as soon as one is on the scene, but until it is, start CPR. (You will learn more about CPR and AED in the following chapters.)

Chapter 3
Answers to Review Questions

1. a
2. b
3. a
4. b
5. c
6. d
7. c
8. c
9. b
10. d

Answers to Scenario

1. The correct answer is c, start CPR beginning with chest compressions. Give CPR to any victim who is in cardiac arrest. Rescue breathing alone is not enough because she does not have a pulse, and you should not waste time calling the dispatcher again. The recovery position is used only for unresponsive victims who are breathing normally and have a pulse.

2. The correct answer is d, cycles of 30 compressions and 2 breaths, with compressions at least 2 inches deep. The ratio of compressions and breaths differs only for two-rescuer CPR for infants and children (15:2). Chest compression depth in a normal-size adult is always at least 2 inches.

3. The correct answer is a, continue with additional cycles of compressions and breaths. Do not interrupt or delay compressions or change the rate of compressions.

4. The correct answer is b, which continues CPR with a smooth transition and no interruptions. Answer choice a would interrupt CPR, making it less effective. Answer choice c is incorrect because compressions and rescue breaths are given at the same time only if an advanced airway has been inserted.

Chapter 4
Answers to Review Questions

1. c
2. b
3. a
4. a
5. d

Answers to Scenario

1. The appropriate first step is b, check for responsiveness and normal breathing. Even though the circumstances seem to indicate he has had a heart attack, do not assume he is not breathing or does not have a pulse. Remember always to perform the initial assessment.

2. The correct answer is c, give CPR starting with chest compressions. The victim is not breathing and has no pulse, so he needs CPR and the AED, but if the AED is not ready, give CPR until it is.

3. The correct answer is d, do not touch the victim during the analysis. The victim should not be disturbed during this time.

4. The appropriate next step is b, continue CPR. This is always done following a shock. You do not need to check for a pulse first. Give 5 cycles of CPR (about 2 minutes) before pausing for the AED to analyze again to determine if another shock is needed.

5. The correct answer is c, put him in the recovery position and monitor his breathing and pulse. Because the victim may again experience cardiac arrest, leave the AED pads in place.

Chapter 5

Answers to Review Questions

1. a

2. c

3. d

4. b

5. a

Answers to Scenario

1. The correct answer is a, give abdominal thrusts because he is a responsive choking victim. You cannot give rescue breathing (if needed) until you clear the airway obstruction. Pounding on the back is generally not an effective technique. CPR is used to clear an airway obstruction in an unresponsive victim.

2. The correct answer is c, make sure help has been called. It is crucial to get more help on the way because he may have only minutes to live if you cannot clear the airway obstruction. Abdominal thrusts are used only for a responsive victim. Rescue breathing would be used only after the obstruction is cleared, assuming the victim is still not breathing. Checking his mouth for a foreign object is done later during CPR.

3. The correct answer is c, give CPR starting with chest compressions. Pounding on his sternum is not an effective technique, and an AED is likely not needed immediately, as his primary problem is choking. Check his mouth only after 30 chest compressions, when you open the mouth to give rescue breaths.

Glossary

A

Abandonment: a type of negligence that occurs if someone who has begun to give care leaves the victim before care is taken over by someone with an equal or higher level of training.

Acquired immunodeficiency syndrome (AIDS): a fatal disease caused by the human immunodeficiency virus (HIV).

Acute myocardial infarction: a condition of dying cardiac muscle tissue caused by sudden reduced blood flow to the heart muscle; also known as heart attack.

Advance directive: a legal document signed by an individual, often a terminally ill person, and his or her doctor, that restricts what medical care the person will accept; a living will.

Advanced cardiac life support (ACLS): medical procedures needed to restore a heartbeat beyond the procedures of basic life support.

Airborne transmission: transmission of a pathogen from one person to another through the air, usually via small fluid droplets the infected person coughs or sneezes out.

Airway: a shaped, tubelike device inserted into the mouth or nose that helps keep a victim's airway open during resuscitation or until the victim receives advanced medical attention.

Airway obstruction: a condition in which the victim's airway is partially or completely obstructed by the tongue, vomit or other body tissue or fluids, or a foreign object; choking.

Angina pectoris: chest pain caused by heart disease; usually occurs after intense activity or exertion; often called angina.

Aspiration: the movement of vomit or other fluids or solids into the lungs.

Atherosclerosis: a narrowing and "hardening" of the arteries caused by plaque.

B

Bag mask or bag-valve-mask (BVM): a resuscitation mask unit connected to a bag that is squeezed to provide air or oxygen to a non-breathing victim.

Barrier device: a device, such as a pocket mask, used to provide a barrier between the victim and the rescuer when giving rescue breathing to reduce the risk of disease transmission.

Basic life support (BLS): emergency care given to a victim with a life-threatening problem of the airway or circulation; generally refers to rescue breathing, CPR and use of an AED.

Bloodborne transmission: transmission of disease from one person to another through contact with the infected person's blood or certain other body fluids.

Brachial pulse: the pulse felt over the brachial artery in an infant's upper arm on the inside, about midway between the shoulder and elbow.

Bronchodilator: an inhaled medication used by people with asthma to prevent or control asthmatic attacks.

C

Call fast: situation in which, when alone with an unresponsive victim, you give 2 minutes of basic life support before pausing to call for help and an AED.

Call first: situation in which, when alone with an unresponsive victim, you call for help and an AED before starting basic life support.

Cardiac arrest: the sudden stop of the heartbeat.

Cardiopulmonary resuscitation (CPR): a basic life support procedure for a victim who is not breathing and has no heartbeat, consisting of rescue breathing combined with chest compressions.

Carotid pulse: the pulse felt over the carotid artery in the neck of an adult or child.

Chain of survival: a concept emphasizing five steps needed for cardiac arrest victims: immediate recognition of the cardiac arrest and activation of the emergency response system, early CPR with emphasis on chest compressions, rapid defibrillation, effective advanced life support and integrated post-cardiac arrest care.

Cholesterol: a fatty substance the body needs to carry out important functions but that at high levels is a risk factor for cardiovascular disease.

Cincinnati Prehospital Stroke Scale (CPSS): a screening process for rapid identification of a stroke outside a hospital setting.

Competent: the victim is able to understand what is happening and the implications of his or her decision to receive or refuse emergency care.

Confidentiality: the general principle that one should not give out any information about a victim to anyone except for those caring for the victim.

Consent: the victim's permission for a trained rescuer to provide emergency care.

Coronary artery disease: blockage of vessels supplying heart muscle with blood, often leading to heart attack.

Critical incident stress debriefing: a formal program in many organizations and facilities to assist those experiencing the effects of stress after an emergency.

D

Decontamination: the use of physical or chemical means to remove, inactivate or destroy bloodborne pathogens on a surface or item so that it is no longer infectious.

Defibrillation: the process of administering an electrical shock to a fibrillating heart to restore a normal heart rhythm.

Direct contact: disease transmission that occurs when someone directly contacts an infected person, or fluids or substances from that person.

Disinfectant: a substance, such as a bleach solution, that kills most pathogens on contaminated surfaces.

Dispatcher: an EMS professional who answers 9-1-1 calls, determines the nature of the emergency, and sends the appropriate emergency personnel to the scene.

Do Not Resuscitate (DNR) order: a specific kind of advance directive that indicates the ill person has chosen not to be resuscitated if his or her heart and breathing stop.

Duty to act: the legal obligation to care for a victim of a medical emergency, accepted as a dimension of a trained professional's job description.

E

Electrodes: the pads of an automated external defibrillator that attach to the main unit with cables and deliver a shock to a victim's chest when indicated.

Emergency medical services (EMS) system: a comprehensive network of professionals linked together to provide appropriate levels of medical care for victims of injury or sudden illness.

Emergency medical responder: formerly called a first responder, a professional with BLS training who often arrives first at the scene of a medical emergency.

Emergency medical technician (EMT): emergency personnel trained to give prehospital medical treatment to injured or ill victims and to transport victims to advanced care facilities.

Engineering controls: devices that isolate or remove the bloodborne pathogen hazard.

EpiPen: a commercially available emergency epinephrine auto-injector for use by those experiencing severe allergic reactions to bee stings, certain foods, etc.

Exposure control plan: a plan employers must have in place to prevent exposure to bloodborne pathogens.

Expressed consent: consent explicitly given by the victim for emergency care.

F

Femoral pulse: the pulse felt in the center of the groin crease.

Fibrillation: an abnormal heart rhythm in which muscles of the heart are quivering instead of beating rhythmically; see ventricular fibrillation.

Flowmeter: a device, usually built into an oxygen pressure regulator, used to adjust the rate of oxygen delivery to the victim.

G

Good Samaritan law: a state law designed to protect people from being sued for giving emergency care.

H

Heimlich maneuver: abdominal thrusts given to a responsive choking victim to expel an obstructing object.

Hepatitis: the various forms of liver disease caused by the bloodborne hepatitis B virus (HBV), hepatitis C virus (HCV), or other hepatitis viruses.

Human immunodeficiency virus (HIV): the virus that causes AIDS.

Hypertension: high blood pressure.

I

Implied consent: consent that a rescuer can assume is given to administer emergency care to an unresponsive victim or a child without a parent or guardian present.

Inadequate breathing: breathing so slow that oxygen levels in the blood are dropping to life-threatening levels.

Indirect contact: disease transmission through contact with contaminated objects, food or drink, droplets in the air, or vectors such as insects.

Initial assessment: a quick first check of the victim for life-threatening problems, involving a check for responsiveness, normal breathing and severe bleeding.

M

Medical direction: the process by which EMS personnel and some professional rescuers are guided in certain medical interventions in the field by a physician.

Meningitis: a contagious viral or bacterial infection of the fluid surrounding the spinal cord and brain.

N

Nasal cannula: nasal prongs that deliver oxygen to breathing victims who do not require a high concentration of oxygen.

Nasopharyngeal airway: a nasal airway inserted through the nose and into the pharynx.

Negligence: a breach of duty, when one has a duty to act, that results in injury or damages to a victim.

Nitroglycerin: a prescription medication for angina and heart attack that increases blood flow through partially restricted coronary arteries.

Nonrebreathing mask: an oxygen delivery device consisting of a mask and a reservoir bag, used with breathing victims.

O

Occupational Exposure to Bloodborne Pathogens Standard: a set of regulations from the Occupational Safety and Health Administration (OSHA) designed to protect employees from exposure to bloodborne disease pathogens.

Oropharyngeal airway: an oral airway inserted through the mouth and into the pharynx.

Oxygen delivery device: a device, such as a face mask or nasal cannula, that provides the flowing oxygen to the victim.

P

Pacemaker: a small electronic device, implanted under the skin in some patients with heart disease, that helps the heart maintain a regular rhythm.

Perfusion: the supply of oxygen to and removal of wastes from the cells and tissues of the body as a result of blood flow through the capillaries.

Personal protective equipment (PPE): barriers such as gloves and resuscitation masks that prevent being exposed to blood and other body fluids when caring for a victim in an emergency or working around potentially infected materials.

Pressure regulator: a device attached to an oxygen tank that reduces the pressure of oxygen to a safe level; includes a gauge showing the pressure remaining within the tank.

Professional rescuer: a trained person who, in either an employment or a volunteer situation, has the responsibility to provide emergency care when needed; in this textbook, the professional rescuer is assumed to be trained to the level of a "health care provider BLS rescuer" by 2010 guidelines.

Pulse: a regular pulsing sensation felt over the victim's artery at the neck (adult or child) or upper arm (infant) that signifies the heart is beating and the victim has circulation.

R

Recovery position: a position used for breathing, unresponsive victims while waiting for help to arrive; the victim is positioned on the side to keep the airway open and allow fluids to drain from the mouth; also called the HAINES recovery position (High Arm IN Endangered Spine).

Rescue breathing: a technique for getting air or oxygen into a non-breathing person's lungs to oxygenate the blood.

Respiratory arrest: a condition in which breathing has completely stopped.

Respiratory distress: a condition in which the victim has difficulty breathing.

Resuscitation: a general term referring to the procedures used in an attempt to restore breathing and/or circulation to a victim.

Resuscitation mask: a device that covers the mouth and nose of non-breathing victims to provide rescue breaths.

Risk factor: anything that makes it more likely that a person will develop a particular disease.

S

Scope of practice: actions one is trained and qualified to perform, such as specific basic life support skills performed by professional rescuers.

Secondary assessment: an assessment performed after determining that the victim does not have life-threatening problems, including obtaining a history and performing a physical examination.

Sharps: any devices or items that may accidentally cut a person handling them, such as needles, scissors, scalpels and broken glassware.

Sinus rhythm: the normal rhythm of the heart.

Standard precautions: a set of safety guidelines for treating all blood and other potentially infectious materials as if known to be contaminated.

Standard of care: how emergency care should be performed; what others with the same training would do in a similar situation.

Sterilize: to use a chemical or physical procedure to destroy all microbial life on an item.

Sternum: the breastbone.

Stoma: a hole in the neck used for breathing that was surgically created as a result of an injury or illness.

Stroke: an interruption of blood flow to a part of the brain; also called a cerebrovascular accident (CVA) or brain attack.

Suction device: a mechanical, electrical, or oxygen-powered device used to clear blood, vomit, and other substances from a victim's airway.

Sudden illness: any medical condition that occurs suddenly and requires emergency care.

Sudden infant death syndrome (SIDS): a condition, whose exact cause is poorly understood, that results in an apparently otherwise healthy infant dying suddenly in its sleep.

Supplemental oxygen: oxygen, usually from a tank, delivered to victims in many emergency situations.

Transient ischemic attack (TIA): a temporary interruption to blood flow in an artery in the brain; sometimes called a mini-stroke tripod position: a position often assumed by a victim with respiratory distress: sitting, leaning forward with hands on knees.

Tuberculosis (TB): a highly contagious airborne disease caused by bacteria.

Universal precautions: safety guidelines for treating blood and certain human body fluids as if they are known to be infectious for bloodborne pathogens; the term is generally being replaced by the term standard precautions.

Vector transmission: transmission of a bloodborne pathogen from an infected person or animal through the bite of a tick, mosquito, or other insect.

Ventricular fibrillation (V-fib): an abnormal heart rhythm, which commonly occurs during heart attacks, in which the ventricles of the heart are quivering instead of beating rhythmically.

Work practice controls: specific methods of working around blood or other infectious material that reduce the risk for disease transmission.

Glossary

Index

9-1-1
  call first/call fast rules for 11, 58, 59
  in chain of survival 11
  summary of basic life support 48

A
ABC order of actions in initial assessment. *See* CAB order of
  actions in initial assessment
Abdominal thrusts 51, 52
Acute myocardial infarction. *See* Heart attack
Adults
  AED use for 43
  call first rule for 11
  chest compressions for 23
  choking care for 52, 53
  CPR for adult or child (two rescuers) 29, 30
  CPR for adults, children and infants (one rescuer) 27, 28
  difference from children and infants 10
  drowning prevention for 35
  suctioning 62
  summary of basic life support 48
Advanced Cardiac Life Support (ACLS) 22
Advanced care in chain of survival 11
Advanced resuscitation 61
  airway adjuncts for 64
  suction devices for 61
  supplemental oxygen for 68
AED. *See* Automated External Defibrillator
Airway
  adjuncts for 64
  nasal 66
  opening 13, 14, 24
  oral 64
  suctioning 61
Airway obstruction 50
  assessing for 12, 50
Alcohol, drowning and 35
Alerts
  chest compressions 29
  rescue breathing 34
  using an AED 43
Anaphylaxis 33
Angina pectoris 22
Answers to review questions and case scenarios 74
Aspiration 27
Aspirin 21
Assessment, victim
  initial 12
  secondary 14
Atherosclerosis 18

Automated External Defibrillator (AED)
  alert for 43
  and CPR 40
  attaching to victim 40
  components of 40
  for children and infants 43
  how it works 40
  in chain of survival 11, 39
  laws for 39
  medical direction for 39
  placement of pads for infants 41
  problems and maintenance 44
  special considerations for 44, 58
  steps for using 40
  summary of basic life support 48
  using an AED 42
  voice and visual prompts from 41

B
Back blows 51, 54
Bag mask (BVM)
  oxygen delivery via 66, 73
  rescue breathing via 26, 66
  single-rescuer use of 68
  two-rescuer use of 68, 69
Barrier devices 24, 25
Basic life support (BLS)
  in emergencies 1
  overview 10
  summary of basic life support 48
Battery, consent and 5
Bleeding, checking for severe 13
Bradycardia
  compressions for infants or children 35
Brachial pulse 13
Bronchodilator 33
Bulb syringe 61

C
CAB order of actions in initial assessment 13
Call first/call fast 11
  for near drowning 59
  for trauma 58
Cardiac arrest
  AED use for 43
  causes of 22
  chain of survival for 11
  CPR for 22
  in children 43
  ventricular fibrillation in 39
Cardiopulmonary Resuscitation (CPR)

Index